Wafa SOUDANI
Mohammed BOUACHRINE
Fatima Zohra HADJADJ-AOUL

Impact of the Covid-19 health crisis on the Algerian population

Wafa SOUDANI
Mohammed BOUACHRINE
Fatima Zohra HADJADJ-AOUL

Impact of the Covid-19 health crisis on the Algerian population

Psychosocial, organic sequelae and diabetes

ScienciaScripts

Contents

Wafa SOUDANI

Lecturer in Therapeutic Chemistry Department of Pharmacy Faculty
of Medicine Annaba
Badji-Mokhtar University Annaba, Algeria

Mohammed BOUACHRINE

Professor of Molecular Chemistry, Faculty of Science, Moulay Ismail
University, Meknes, Morocco.

Fatima Zohra HADJADJ-AOUL

Professor of Therapeutic Chemistry Department of Pharmacy Faculty
of Medicine Algiers Ben Youcef Ben Khedda University Algiers,
Algeria

To all my loved ones.

Sante et gaiete, donnent la beaute Health and gaiety, give beauty
Salud y alegna, hermosura cria.
Spanish proverb
Wafa SOUDANI

FOREWORD

Sars-CoV-2 is a new virus in the coronavirus family; discovered in China in December 2019, it has gradually led to a pandemic since March 2020. It generally causes a mild infectious syndrome, but can also lead to serious clinical symptoms and sometimes death. Algeria, like many other countries around the world, is also affected by this scourge, which has introduced a wide range of health problems. The Algerian government has put in place a number of preventive measures to curb the spread of the virus.

The Covid-19 pandemic has had a major impact on health systems, the economy, education and daily life in many countries. Measures such as lockdowns, business closures and travel restrictions have been put in place to limit the damage caused by this health problem. Since the start of the pandemic, Algeria has reported a significant number of cases of Covid-19, in addition to a complex acute presentation that can affect several organ systems; there is considerable evidence to suggest that long-term sequelae are common and far-reaching; it is in this context that the present work is set.

The publication of this book is intended to alleviate the problem of the lack of data on the risk of the Covid19 pandemic in Algeria, the Maghreb countries and Europe. This book is designed to meet the following objectives

Assessing the organic and psychosocial sequelae of coronavirus infection in the Algerian population.

Assessing the relationship between the Covid-19 pandemic and diabetes.

Compare the frequency of the long Covid between men and women.

This manuscript deals with a descriptive and integrated survey in six 6 chapters enlivened by 80 figures and 50 illustrative tables in the medical and pharmaceutical fields.

We hope that reading this work will provide answers to the questions of researchers in the field of microbiology and infectiology, and that it will satisfy the scientific curiosity of colleagues in medicine and pharmacy.

We would like to thank all the people who, from near or far, contributed to the revision and expertise of this book, especially the Dean of the Faculty of Medicine Annaba Pr. AMOURA Kamel, and President of the Scientific Council Pr. MELLOUKI Youcef.

Our sincere thanks go to the Heads of the Department of Pharmacy, Professor MERRICHE Hacene, and to all the teachers at the Faculty of Medicine in Annaba. In particular, we would like to thank them for their unconditional support during my university hospital career at the Faculty of Medicine in Annaba, Algeria.

The authors would like to thank all those who collaborated in the distribution and publication of this book, in particular the Head of the Library Department, Mme CHAIB Nora, Mme BOUDERBALA Sihem, and Mme REDJIMI Wahida.

Wafa SOUDANI
e-mail. wafa24soud@gmail.com.
E-learning link: https://elearning.univ-annaba.dz/user/profile.php?id=3245
ORCID-ID. http://orcid.org/0000-0003-2125-2701
ResearchGate: https://www.researchgate.net/profile/Wafa-Soudani

Introduction

The coronavirus pandemic (Covid-19) has spread very rapidly to cover 210 countries and territories around the world. Sars-CoV-2 began in Wuhan, China, in December 2019. The agent causing the infection was rapidly detected as a beta coronavirus; initially named new coronavirus (2019-nCoV). It probably originated from bat-derived coronaviruses that spread via an intermediate mammalian host to humans. The Sars-CoV-2 viral genome was rapidly sequenced to enable diagnostic tests, epidemiological monitoring and the development of preventive and therapeutic strategies.

The severity of the disease can vary from person to person, ranging from mild to more severe forms that may require hospitalisation and intensive care. Older people and those with underlying health problems, such as cardiovascular, pulmonary or immune disorders, are more likely to develop serious complications.

However, the disappearance of the pandemic did not mark the end of the health crisis caused by Covid 19; rather, it left the world with mild to severe after-effects. These after-effects were later referred to as "Covid long" or "post-Covid-19 syndrome".

The sequelae of Covid-19 are the effects or symptoms that persist or last for several weeks or even months. These may occur after infection with the Sars-CoV-2 virus, which causes the disease. These symptoms can vary considerably from one person to another and can affect different systems in the body.

The objectives of our research are :

Primary objective

•   Assessing the organic and psychosocial sequelae of coronavirus infection in the Algerian population.

Secondary objectives

•   Assessing the relationship between Covid-19 and diabetes.

•   Compare the frequency of long covid between men and women.

Chapter I

History

History

The coronavirus family causes respiratory infections in mammals and birds. They are RNA viruses divided into four sub-families: Alphacoronavirus, Betacoronavirus, Gammacoronavirus and Deltacoronavirus. In humans, four are responsible for benign pathologies in immunocompetent patients (HCoV-229E, HCoV-OC43, HCoV-NL63 and HKU1). [1]

Two are responsible for serious and potentially fatal diseases: SARS-CoV-1 and MERS-CoV, identified in 2003 and 2012 respectively. [2] [3]

Sars-CoV-1 was responsible for 774 deaths in 2002-2003 after infecting 8096 people, mainly in China's Guangdong province and Hong Kong. The fatality rate was estimated at 9.6%. Ten years later, MERS-CoV caused a localised epidemic in the Middle East. The rate of illness was estimated at 38%. In 2015, a second epidemic occurred in South Korea, resulting in 36 deaths out of 186 confirmed cases. [4]

The origin of these two viruses was zoonotic: Sars-CoV-1 may have spread to humans from civets, raccoons or ferrets [5] and MERS-CoV from dromedaries. [6] The natural host in both cases was the bat. [1]

At the end of December 2019, the appearance of several cases of pneumonia of unknown origin in Hubei in China led to the identification, in January 2020, of a new coronavirus [7], called Sars-CoV-2 by the Coronavirus Working Group of the International Committee on Taxonomy of Viruses [8]. It is a Beta-coronavirus probably transmitted to humans by pangolins at the Huanan seafood market in Wuhan [9].

Human-to-human transmission led to the virus spreading to Thailand and then to other countries, causing a pandemic today, while the exact route of infection of the first case remains uncertain. [10]

Chapter II

General information about Covid-19

II.1. Epidemiological data

II.1.1. Origin and development

The number of Covid-19 cases reported to the WHO has been steadily increasing since the first report of Covid-19 in December 2019 by the WHO country office in China. [11]

A. In China:

China is the country on the Asian continent that has seen the largest outbreak of Covid-19. Between 3 January 2020 and 6 May 2023, a total of 99,261,812 confirmed cases of Covid-19 were reported in China.

were notified, of which 121,144 died. [12]

B. Worldwide :

The Covid-19 pandemic spread in early December 2019 from Wuhan, and was then exported to a growing number of countries. By 2 March 2020, outside China, 67 territories had reported 8565 confirmed cases of Covid-19 with 132 deaths [13], as well as significant community spread occurring in several countries around the world. Following the rapid spread and acceleration of cases worldwide, the WHO declared Covid-19 a pandemic on 11 March 2020. [14] Worldwide, as of 16 May 2023, 766,895,075 confirmed cases and more than 69,358,889 deaths have been notified to the WHO. [15]

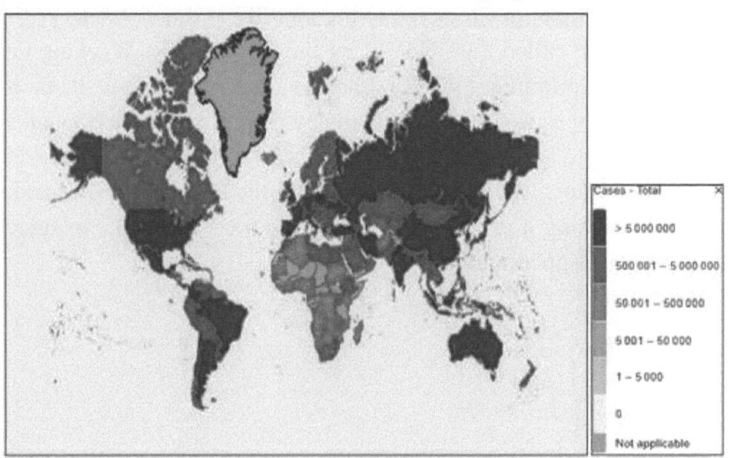

Figure 1: World map showing countries with confirmed cases of Sars-CoV-2 in May 2023. [15]

C. Europe :

In May 2023, the main endemic outbreaks were concentrated in the United

Kingdom (24,611066 cases/225,852 deaths), Italy (25,842,595 cases/190,242 deaths), and Spain (13,868,22 cases/121,213 deaths). The rest of Europe is also affected by the coronavirus epidemic: Russia (22,917,873 cases/398,919 deaths) and Germany (38,423,300 cases/174,032 deaths). [15]

D. In France :

In May 2023, there had been 39,010,097 confirmed cases and 163,437 deaths linked to the coronavirus since the start of the epidemic. [15]

E.The Greater Maghreb :

The Greater Maghreb recorded its first confirmed cases between 25 February 2020 in Algeria and 13 March in Mauritania, followed by Tunisia and Morocco.

•   In Algeria

The number of confirmed cases has risen steadily since the first case was reported on 25 February 2020 in the wilaya of Ouargla. At present, the total number of confirmed cases of Covid-19 in Algeria is 271,820, and the total number of deaths is

by Covid-19 is 6,881 [15].

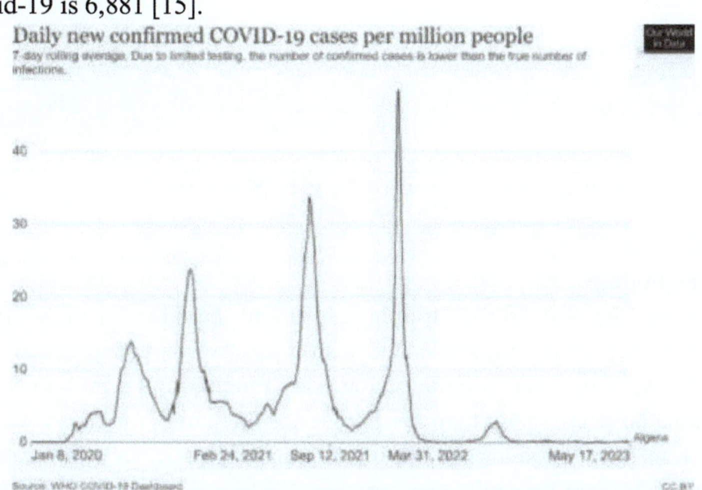

Figure 2: New confirmed daily cases of Covid-19 per million population in Algeria. [16]

•   Tunisia

There have been 1,153,161 cases of contamination and 29,412 deaths linked to the coronavirus.

recorded in the country since the start of the pandemic. [15]

•   Morocco

The total number of confirmed Covid-19 cases is 1,274,180, with 16,297 deaths recorded in the country since the start of the pandemic. [15]

• Libya:

In Libya, there have been 507,255 confirmed cases of the coronavirus and 6,437 deaths since the start of the pandemic. [15]

II.2. Sars-cov-2

II.2.1. Taxonomy

Sars is an infectious disease caused by Sars-CoV, a member of the coronavirus family (table 1).

Table 1: Classification and taxonomy, genome and size of human coronaviruses (HCoV) [17]

Human coronavirus (HCoV)

Order: Nidovirales	
Family: Coronaviridae	
Subfamily: Coronavirinae	
Genres : Alphacoronaviruses: HCov-229E and HCoV-NL63 Betacoronavirus : Clade A: HCoV-OC43 and HCoV-HKU1 Clade B: SARS-CoV Clade C: MERS-CoV	
Genome: single-stranded, positively polarised RNA; 26 to 32 kb.	**Size:** 80 to 200 nm

II.2.2. Morphology

Coronaviruses are enveloped, roughly spherical particles with a diameter ranging from 80 to 200 nm, associated with a positive, non-segmented, single-stranded RNA, have a nucleoprotein, a capsid, a matrix and a protein S (spike) which form a large crown on their surface, hence the Latin prefix *corona*. [18]

The important viral proteins are the nucleocapsid protein (N), the membrane glycoprotein (M) and the spike glycoprotein (S). Sars-CoV-2 differs from other coronaviruses by encoding an additional glycoprotein that possesses acetylesterase and hemagglutination (HE) properties. [19]

A.

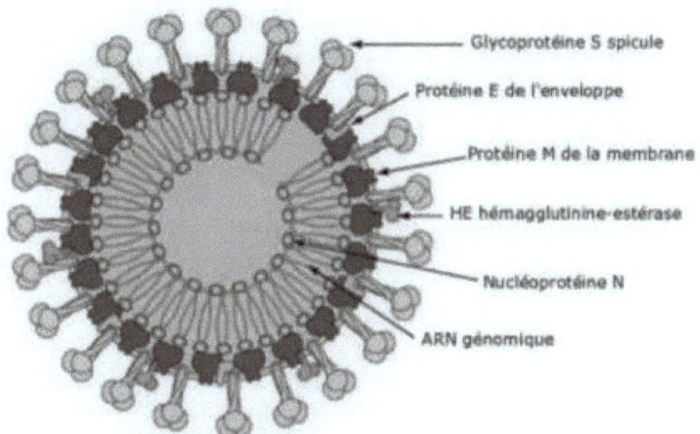

B.

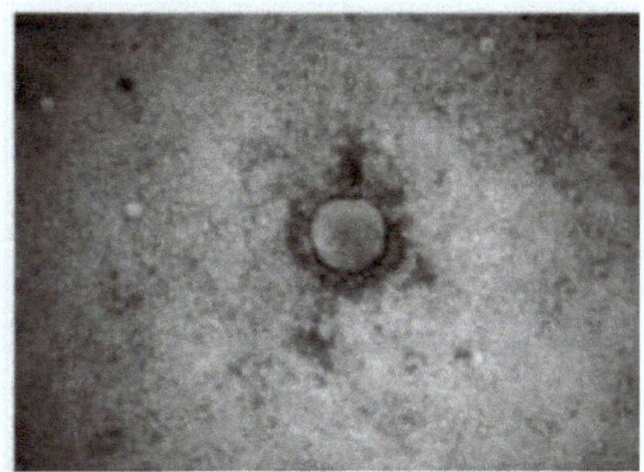

Figure 3: Appearance of coronavirus infectious particles.

A.   Schematic representation of the structure of the coronavirus. [20]
B.   Transmission electron microscopy micrographs of SARS-CoV-2 viral particles. [17]

II.2.3. Covid-19 genome

With a genome size of between 27 and 32 kpb, it is one of the largest RNA viruses known. The Sars-CoV-2 genome comprises around 30,000 nucleotides organised into specific genes encoding structural proteins and non-structural proteins (Nsps). Structural proteins include spike (S), envelope (E), membrane (M) and nucleocapsid (N) proteins. The genomic structure of coronaviruses contains at least six open reading frames (ORFs) [21]. The first ORFs (ORF1a/b) are located at the 5' end, about two-thirds of the total genome length, and code for a poly-protein 1 a and b (pp1a, pp1b). Other ORFs located at the 3' end code for at least four structural proteins:

- The surface glycoprotein (S), responsible for recognising host cell receptors.
- Membrane proteins (M), responsible for shaping virions.
- Envelope proteins (E), responsible for the assembly and release of virions.
- Nucleocapsid (N) proteins are involved in genome packaging of RNA and

virions and play a role in pathogenesis as inhibitors of interferon (IFN).

In addition to the four main structural proteins, there are species-specific structural and accessory proteins, such as HE, 3a/b and 4a/b. [22]

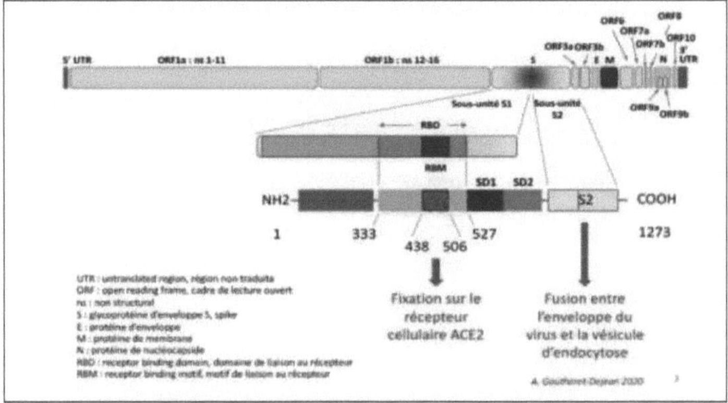

Figure 4: Schematic structure of Sars-CoV-2 gënomic RNA and the Spike protein. [23]

II.2.4. Virus reservoir

The origin of Sars-CoV-2 has not yet been fully determined. However, the results of the genomic analysis of the new virus show a 96.2% similarity with that of a coronavirus linked to bat Sars (Sars-CoV; RaTG13) collected in the Yunnan region of China. This genetic similarity of Sars-CoV-2 and RaTG13 indicates that bat-derived Sars- CoV-2. [24]

Competing evidence has also proposed pangolins as a potential intermediate species for the emergence of Sars-CoV-2. This suggests that pangolins as a potential reservoir species. [25]

Chapter III

Sars-CoV-2 infection

III.1. Transmission mode

The virus is transmitted mainly by respiratory droplets. They are loaded with viral particles which could infect a susceptible subject either by direct contact with a mucous membrane (direct transmission), or by contact with an infected surface via the nasal, buccal or conjunctival mucous membranes (indirect transmission). [26]

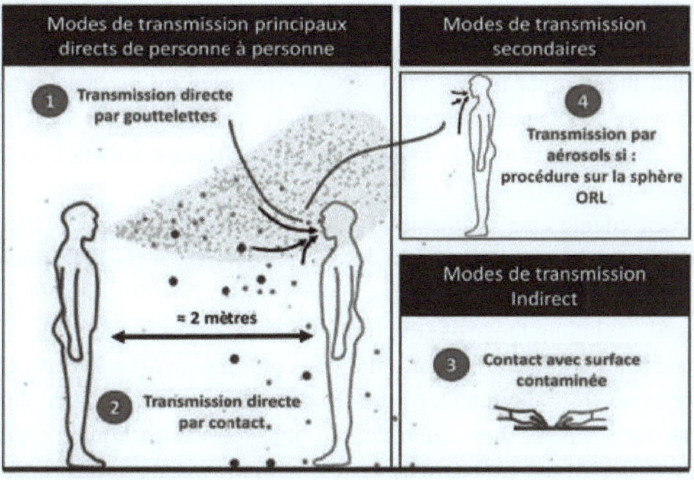

Figure 5: Schematic representation of the different modes of transmission of Sars-CoV-2. [27]

The fecal-oral route was mentioned very early on as a possible route of transmission of Covid-19, and Sars-CoV-2 viral RNA has also been detected in the faeces of patients with Covid-19. [28]

The ocular surface is also a possible transmission route for Sars-COV-2. In addition, expression of ACE2 and TMPRSS has been detected in the conjunctiva, limbus and cornea, making the eye a potential entry point for Sars-COV-2. [29]

III.2 Sars-CoV-2 cycle

One of the main determinants of the initiation and progression of Sars-CoV-2 infection is viral entry into host cells. In the endosomal pathway, clathrin-dependent endocytosis and enzymatic cleavage of protein S represent two critical steps in the process of virus entry and host cell infection.

The life cycle of Sars-CoV-2 takes between 8 and 10 hours to complete:
- Attachment to the host cell's plasma membrane,
- Intracellular penetration of the virus,
- Expression of the replicase enzyme,
- Replication and transcription of viral RNA and assembly and release of virions.

After activation of protein S by cleavage by the cellular transmembrane protease serine 2 (TMPRSS2) into S1 and S2 subunits, S1 binds to the ACE2 receptor via the receptor binding domain (RBD) and, more specifically, the receptor binding motif (RBM). S2 allows fusion between the plasma membrane and the viral envelope. [23]

The viral particles enter the cell by endocytosis. Following fusion of the viral envelope with the membrane of the endocytosis vesicle, the nucleocapsid is released into the cytoplasm and viral RNA is released by decapsidation. ORF1 and ORF1ab are translated into poly-proteins 1a and 1ab, which are cleaved by ORF1a proteases to form the RNA replicase-transcriptase complex made up of 16 non-structural proteins.

This complex enables the synthesis of RNA of negative polarity, which serves as a template for the synthesis of new genomic RNAs of positive polarity and subgenomic messenger RNAs. During transcription, 7 to 9 subgenomic RNAs are produced, including those of structural proteins.

The nucleocapsid is assembled from the new genome and the N capsid protein. New virions bud from the lumen of the Golgi apparatus and are then directed to the cell surface where they are released into the extracellular medium by exocytosis, fusion of the endocytosis vesicle with the plasma membrane. [23]

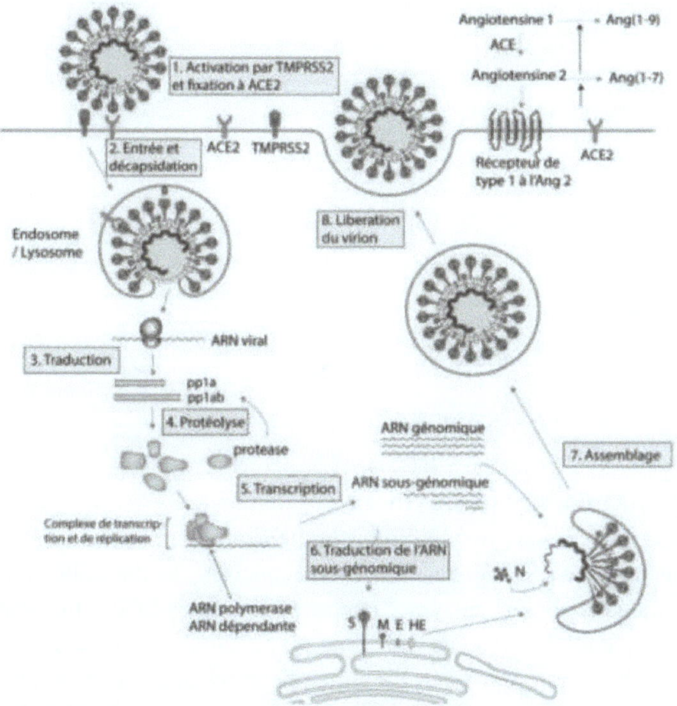

Figure 6: Sars-CoV-2 replication cycle. [26]

III.3. Covid-19 phases

Covid-19 appears to pass through three successively more severe phases (Figure 7) [30]. The first phase (Γ precocious infection) lasts from the time of virus contraction until a few days after the onset of symptoms. It lasts 7 to 10 days and is dominated by significant reproduction of the virus in the upper and lower airways, with predominantly viral symptoms (fever and cough) [31]. The second phase (pulmonary involvement) is characterised by the onset of inflammation and the development of viral pneumonia without hypoxia (IIA), then with hypoxia (IIB) following dyspnoea. The third and final phase is known as hyperinflammation. It is marked by a systemic inflammatory response syndrome with an increased risk of development of acute respiratory distress syndrome (ARDS) and the occurrence of thromboembolic events following hypercoagulability of the blood [30].

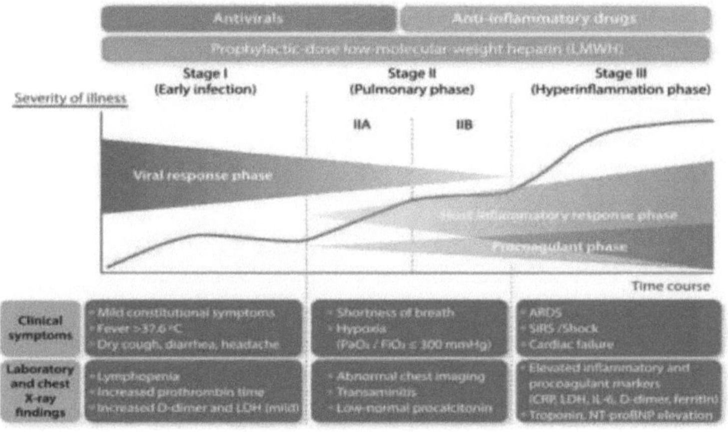

Figure 7: Covid-19 phases [30].

III.4. Pathophysiology of Covid 19

When inhaled, the coronavirus multiplies in the epithelium of the upper airways by attaching itself, via its Spike protein-like spicules, to the cellular receptor ACE-2, a transmembrane enzyme exposed on the surface of respiratory epithelial cells, endothelial cells and type II pneumocytes in the pulmonary alveoli. From the respiratory tract, the virus disperses and infects several other organs, targeting cells expressing this same receptor. The viral load will consequently be increased at the expense of cell survival. [32,33]

During the first phase of the disease (5 to 7 days after infection), the virus is confronted by innate immunity, which attempts to isolate it and limit its spread before the adaptive immune response arrives.

Firstly, when replicating inside host cells, the virus is recognised by intracellular Toll-like receptors (TLRs) 3, 7, 8, RIG-1 and MDA5. This recognition induces the production of IFN-1 by infected alveolar tissue cells and immune plasmacytoid dendritic cells. IFN-1 is an innate pro-inflammatory cytokine that plays a major role in viral clearance through its ability to reprogram cells into an antiviral state. [34, 35]

At the same time, chemokines used to recruit certain leukocytes and pro-inflammatory cytokines are produced, acting as a second layer of the antiviral response. [36]

Around the 7th day after the start of infection, the orchestra of the immune response is mainly represented by the cells of adaptive immunity. The TH1-type immune response mediated by cytotoxic TCD8 lymphocytes specific for viral proteins, in particular spike proteins, is the body's crucial weapon in the defence against Sars-CoV- 2. Their major role is to destroy all infected cells by apoptosis. Active B lymphocytes participate by producing neutralising antibodies directed against the spike protein.

As for TCD4 lymphocytes, their role in modulating the immune response is ensured by the secretion of cytokines. [23,35]

In the majority of cases (85%), this immune response eliminates the virus in seven to ten days, resulting in recovery with a moderate inflammatory response: the infection is therefore benign.

However, the immune response may be inadequate in some patients, who develop severe forms with respiratory distress and sometimes death. Around day 6-7eme , an intense inflammatory response appears, even though the viable virus has usually disappeared, with massive production of cytokines ("cytokine storm") by immune cells infiltrating the tissues, leading to pulmonary redeme and thrombo-embolic disorders, culminating in often fatal multivisceral failure.

111.5. Symptoms of Covid 19

Covid-19 initially causes the classic symptoms of a respiratory infection: fever and cough. The infection can also cause viral lung damage, resulting in respiratory gene (dyspnea).

Other signs may accompany or replace these, but less systematically: muscle pain (myalgia), headaches (cephalea), sore throat, nasal congestion, nausea, vomiting, diarrhoea, etc. The sudden onset of a loss of taste (agueusia) or smell (anosmia) in the absence of rhinitis is also one of the most discriminating signs for suspecting Covid-19. Dermatologically, some people develop erythema (redness) or a rash, and more rarely frostbite, particularly on the toes[37].

111.6. Methods for detecting Sars-CoV-2

A. Polymerase Chain Reaction (PCR)

The diagnostic method of choice for Sars-CoV-2 is genomic detection using a molecular biology method (Reverse Transcription-Polymerase Chain Reaction or RT-PCR) in respiratory samples, preferably a nasopharyngeal swab. RT-PCR is highly specific, with a sensitivity of between 95% and 97% [38]. However, false negative results may occur, especially if the test is performed at the very beginning or end of the viral infection. [39]

B. Serological tests

It consists of detecting IgM and IgG antibodies directed specifically against Sars-CoV-2, either by rapid chromatographic immunoassays or by conventional enzyme immunoassay methods. [38]

These tests are carried out on blood samples and used to identify patients who have developed immunity to the virus.

Seroconversion is rapid, with IgM usually detectable from the onset of symptoms and IgG 10 to 14 days later. [38]

C. Rapid antigen tests

The principle is generally based on immuno-chromatography, with reading either manual or automated. Their main advantage is the rapid turnaround time for results.

15 to 30 minutes. However, its sensitivity is inferior to that of PCR, which is why it is nevertheless being considered for screening contagious individuals with a high viral load. [39]

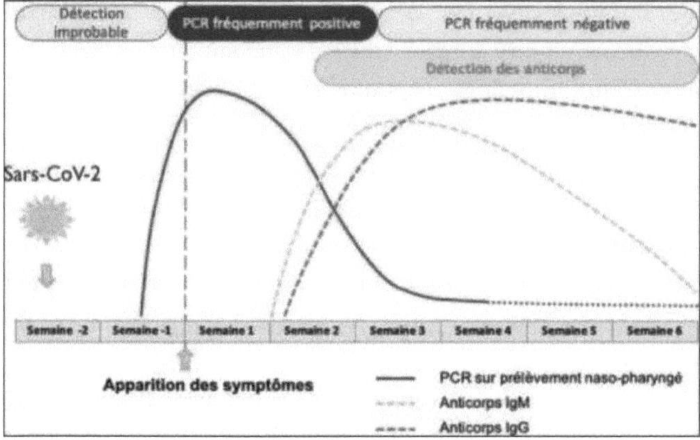

Figure 8: Kinetics of diagnostic markers according to stage of infection.

Chapter IV

Treatment and therapeutic strategy against Sars-CoV-2

^.1. Medical treatment

All stages of the virus life cycle are potential targets for Covid-19 treatment (figure 9). [40]

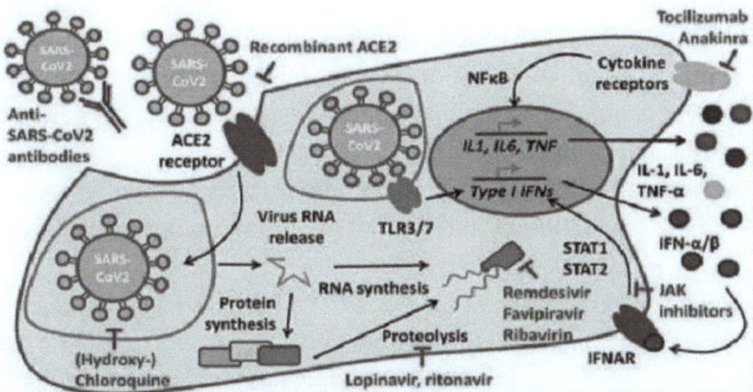

Figure 9: Targets for drugs used in the management of Covid-19. [41]

IV.1.1. Antimalarial drugs

A. Hydroxychloroquine

• Chemical structure

Hydroxychloroquine is a racemic mixture consisting of an R and S enantiomer. Hydroxychloroquine is an aminoquinoline like chloroquine. It was developed during the Second World War as a derivative of Quinacrine with less severe side effects. [42]

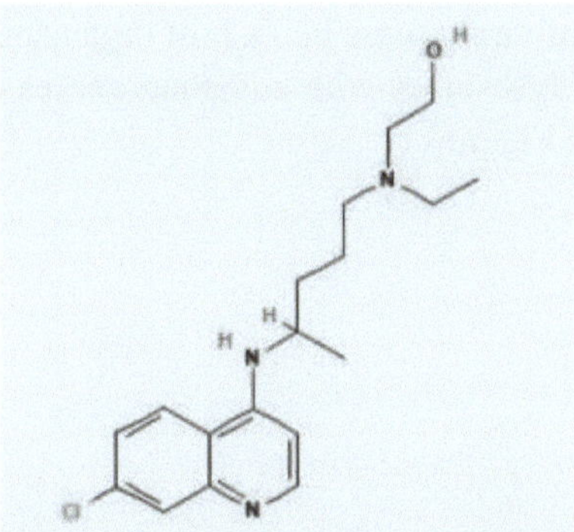

Figure 10: 2D structure of the molecule. [43]

- IUPAC name: 2-[4-[(7-chloroquinolin-4-yl)amino]pentyl-ethylamino] ethanol [43]
- Molecular formula: Ci8H$_{26}$ ClN$_3$ O [42]
- Relationship between chemical structure and therapeutic activity

The amine nitrogen attached to the chloroquine moiety is responsible for the fundamental nature of the drug. There is no major role for the secondary alkyl group attached with the carbon next to the amine group near the chloroquine moiety. The tertiary amine in the terminal position is very important for the activity of the drug. The size of the space between the terminal nitrogen and the 4-amino group is sensitive to the resistance of the parasite. Compounds with shorter or longer chains retain activity against resistant species of parasite.

- Therapeutic indications

Hydroxychloroquine is indicated for the prophylaxis of malaria where resistance to Chloroquine is not reported, the treatment of uncomplicated malaria (caused by

P. *falciparum*, P. *malariae*, P. *ovale or P. vivax*), chronic discoid lupus erythematosus, disseminated lupus erythematosus, rheumatoid arthritis ждиё and chronic rheumatoid arthritis. [42] -WHO recommendations

The WHO does not recommend the use of Hydroxychloroquine as a treatment for Covid-19, as it has not reduced either mortality or the need for, or duration of, artificial ventilation. However, it may increase the risk of cardiac arrhythmia, blood and lymphatic disorders, kidney damage and liver disorders and failure. [44] - Mode of action

HCQ has demonstrated its potential to destroy Sars-CoV-2 in fagons: -Inhibition by interference in the endocytic pathway: [45]

HCQ collects in endosomes and lysosomes and leads to pH neutralisation, which hampers the effects of proteases, preventing protein S cleavage and, ultimately, the process of viral access into a host organism.

HCQ inhibits fusion of lysosomes with autophagosomes due to deregulation of syntaxin 17 as shown in Figure 11.

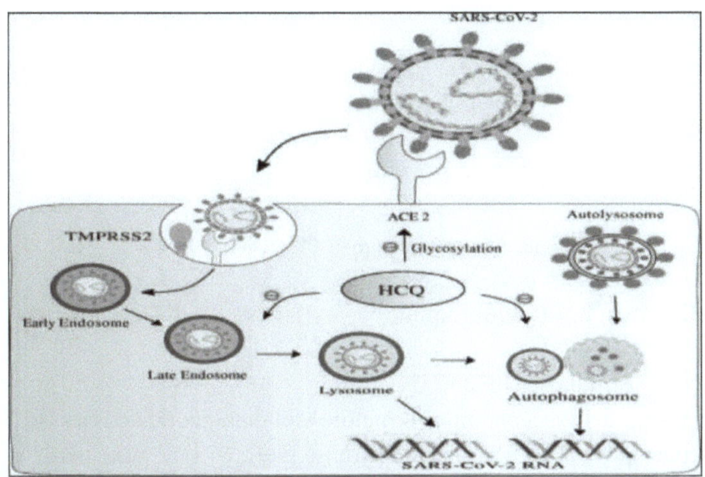

Figure 11: Mechanism of action of hydroxy chloroquine. [45]

-Inhibition by blocking sialic acid receptors :

Recently, it has been identified that the N-terminus of the S protein in Sars-CoV-2 is similar to the region where binding to sialic acid receptors occurs in MERS-CoV. Therefore, Sars-CoV-2 can mediate its entry via these sialic acid receptors in the upper respiratory tract and the previously known ACE2 receptor. Both CQ/HCQ were effective at inhibiting sialic acid, but HCQ was more potent. -Inhibition by preventing cytokine tempetition:

In antigen-presenting cells (APCs), HCQ inhibits antigen processing and presentation to T lymphocytes. For this reason, levels of active T lymphocytes decrease, leading to a reduction in the production of cytokines generated by T and B lymphocytes.

The change in pH caused by Hydroxychloroquine also affects the function of the Toll-like receptor (TLR).

8. Chloroquine

- Chemical structure

Chloroquine is derived from aminoquinoline, the quinoline of which is substituted in position 4 by a [5-(diethylamino)pentan-2-yl]amino group and in position 7 by h chlorine. It also has a broad-spectrum antiviral effect. [46]

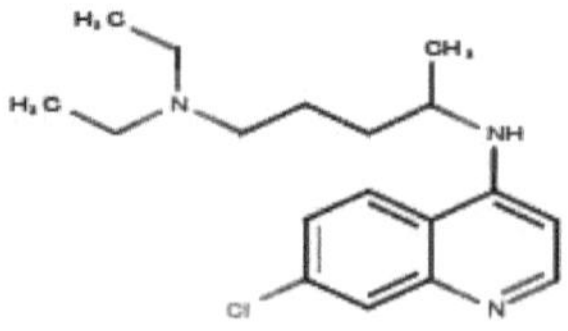

Figure 12: 2D structure of Chloroquine. [47]

- IUPAC name: 4-N-(7-chloroquinolin-4-yl)-1-N,1-N-diethylpentane-1,4-diamine [48]
- Molecular formula: C18H26C1N3 [48]
- Relationship between chemical structure and therapeutic activity

The presence of two basic nitrogen atoms, pka1 = 10.2 and pka2 = 8.1, is essential to the expression of its biological activity. The chlorine atom attached to the quinoline nucleus in position 7 is a key element in biological activity. Substitution by a hydrogen atom results in a drop of more than 90% in its antimalarial properties. [49]

- Indication

It is mainly used in the curative treatment of malaria attacks, except in cases of chloroquine resistance [52]. Chloroquine is also used off-label for the treatment of rheumatic diseases, as well as the treatment and prophylaxis of the Zika virus. [47]

- Mode of action

- Inhibition of endocytosis and alkalinisation of lysosomes :

The effect of Chloroquine against Sars-Cov-2 is: a general reduction in the capacity of cells to carry out clathrin-mediated endocytosis and the prevention of endosome-lysosome fusion, thus preventing the recycling of membrane receptors, which is considered necessary for the cellular entry of Sars-Cov-2. Chloroquine is a weak base that increases lysosomal pH, thereby inhibiting glycosylation[50].

-Inhibition of viral transcription by binding to Uracile and Adenine nucleotides. [50]

❖ **Association of zinc and Chloroquine**

The role of zinc in Rdrp inhibition: Chloroquine increases zinc absorption into cells and stimulates its intracellular accumulation.

Zn ions^{2+} inhibit transcription of viral mRNAs; the activity of the nsp12 Rdrp subunit of Sars-CoV; the activity of the nsp14 subunit, which is responsible for correcting transcription errors during elongation, by forming bonds with it and changing its conformation, thus losing its corrective function. [50]

^.1.2. Antibiotherapy

In patients with confirmed Sars-CoV-2 infection, there is no indication to
prescribe or continue antibiotic therapy in the absence of a documented bacterial
infection. [51]

A. Special case of Azithromycin :

Azithromycin is a macrolide, a subclass of azalides.

It is a derivative of erythromycin A with a nitrogen atom in the ring
lactone. [52]

- Gross formula: $C_{38}H_{72}N_2O_{12}$ [53]
- IUPAC nomenclature: 9-deoxy-9a-aza-9a-methyl-9a homoerythromycin A.
[53]
- Chemical structure

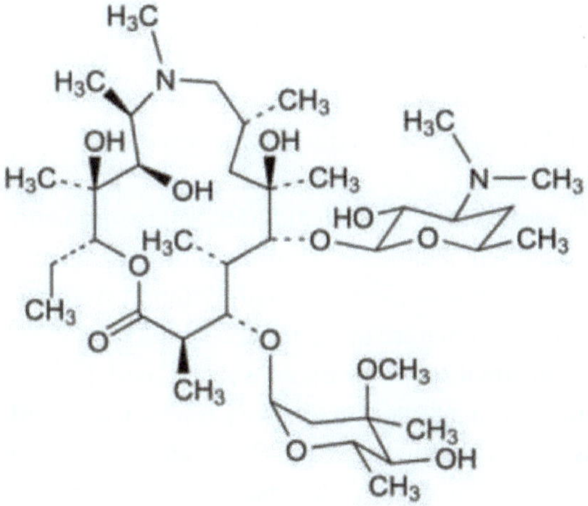

Figure 13: chemical structure of Azithromycin. [53]

- Mode of action

Azithromycin inhibits protein synthesis by reversible binding to the 50S Subunit
of the ribosome at the P site (nascent polypeptide chain). It prevents
translocation of the peptidyl-tRNA complex from the P site to the A site by
This prevents elongation of the peptide chain, blocking the reunion of the last
stage of synthesis by steric hindrance.

- The antiviral activity of Azithromycin (AZ) :

Endosome maturation and function require an acidic environment. AZ is a weak
base and accumulates preferentially intracellularly in lysosomes, which could
increase pH levels and potentially block endocytosis and/or viral gene excretion
from lysosomes, thereby limiting viral replication.

A potential role for AZ in interfering with viral entry via a binding interaction between the Sars-CoV-2 spike protein and the host receptor protein ACE2. [54]

• Immunomodulating properties :

Macrolides can lower inflammatory responses and reduce the excessive production of cytokines associated with respiratory viral infections. It leads to a reduction in the accumulation of leucocytes in the lung tissue and bronchoalveoli, with a large reduction in the number of neutrophils. This reduction in inflammation is independent of changes in viral load. [55]

• Relationship between chemical structure and therapeutic activity

The dimethyl group of the di-methyl amino substituent chain on the sugar amine is the site of metabolism and ribosomal binding. The methyl groups are essential for the hydrogen bonds between the erythromycin A molecule and the amino acids of the 50S ribosomal subunit. The deletion of the cetone function at C9 makes Azithromycin stable in an acidic environment.

• Indication

Azithromycin is used in the treatment of respiratory infections such as influenza or in certain respiratory diseases as adjuvant therapy. [56]

B. Other antibiotics

The French High Council for Public Health (HCSP) recommends :

• No antibiotic treatment should be prescribed for patients presenting symptoms associated with a confirmed Covid-19 (apart from another infectious site), given the exceptional nature of bacterial co-infection.

• That pending confirmation of the diagnosis of Covid-19 :

If there is any doubt about an upper respiratory tract bacterial infection, the recommendations for management (SPILF 2011) should be followed:

- Maxillary sinusitis: Amoxicillin (Pristinamycin if allergic to betalactamins)

- Frontal/ethmoidal/sphenoidal sinusitis: Amoxicillin-Clavulanic acid(Levofloxacin if true allergy to Betalactam)

- Bacterial angina: Amoxicillin (macrolide if truly allergic)

If there is any doubt about a bacterial infection of the lower respiratory tract, the recommendations for management (AFSSAPS 2010) should be followed:

J Healthy subjects: Amoxicillin (Pristinamycin if true allergy)

J Subject with comorbidity(ies) :   Amoxicillin-Acid clavulanic acid (Pristinamycin if really allergic)

J Subject with signs of seriousness: injectable 3eme generation cephalosporin combined with a macrolide. [51]

- Amoxicillin :

• Gross formula: $C_{16}H_{19}N_3O_5S$ [53]

• IUPAC nomenclature: (2S,5 R,6 R)-6-[[(2R)-2-amino- 2-(4-

hydroxyphenyl)acetyl]amino] acid -3,3-dimethyl-7 -oxo-4-thia-1 -
azabicyclo[3.2.0]heptane-2- carboxylic acid. [53]
* Chemical structure :

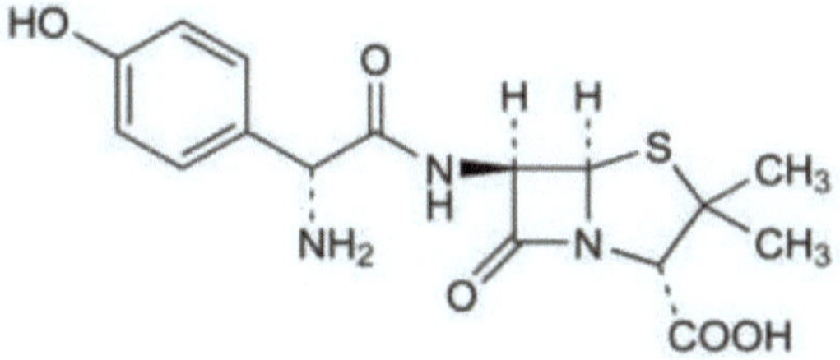

Figure 14: chemical structure of Amoxicillin. [53]

* Mode of action :
Amoxicillin is a broad-spectrum aminopenicillin with bactericidal activity on
young germs in the process of developing their cell wall. It binds to penicillin-
binding proteins (PLPs) located on the inner membrane of the bacterial cell wall
and inactivates them. [57]
Amoxicillin has a structural analogy between the 0-lactam ring and the D-
alanine-D-alanine terminal dipeptide of the peptidoglycan pentapeptide. Their
recognition by transpeptidases and carboxypeptidases (PLP) results in the
attachment of the 0-lactam ring.
on the active site of these target enzymes, which contains a serine. This binding
leads to the opening of the 0-lactam ring by breaking the amide bond and
acylation of the serine active site, with the formation of a covalent penicilloyl-
enzyme complex that results in the inactivation of the enzyme's active site,
thereby inhibiting peptidoglycan synthesis and halting bacterial growth. [58]
- Relationship between chemical structure and therapeutic activity
The integrity of the beta-lactam cycle is essential for activity.
Compliance with the 2S,5R,6R configuration
The acid function in position 2 is important and R1 modifies the
Pharmacokinetics
The R radical plays an important role in intrinsic bacterial activity.

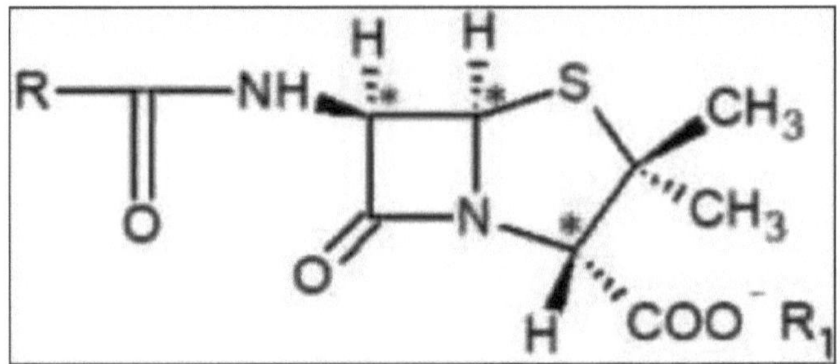

Figure 15: chemical structure of Penicillin.

^.1.3. Antivirals

A. Remdesivir :

Remdesivir is an antiviral previously developed for Ebola virus disease. It was granted European marketing authorisation (MA) on 16 December 2021 for the treatment of Covid-19 disease in adults requiring oxygen therapy with an increased risk of progression to a severe form of Covid-19. [59]

* Gross formula: C27H35N6O8P [60]
* IUPAC nomenclature: 2-ethylbutyl(2S)-2-[[[(2R,3 S,4 R,5R)-5-(4- aminopyrrolo[2,1-f][1,2,4]triazin-7-yl)-5-cyano-3,4-dihydroxyoxolan-2-yl]methoxy phenoxyphosphoryl]amino]propanoate. [60]
* Chemical structure :

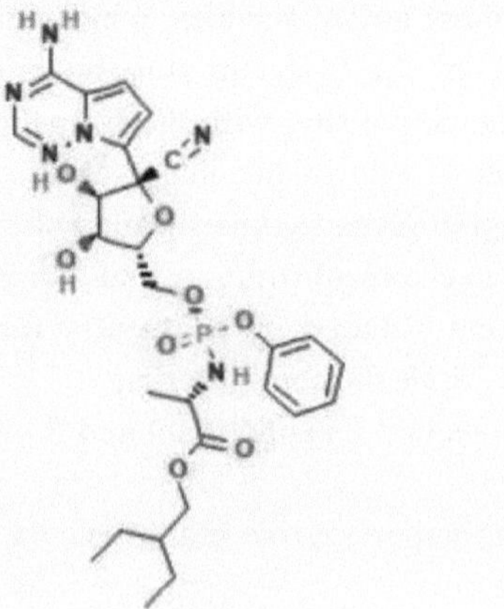

Figure 16: chemical structure of Remdesivir. [60

- Mode of action

It is a prodrug nucleotide analogue of adenosine whose triphosphate inhibits Sars-CoV-2 RNA polymerase by competition. [52]

Remdesivir acts as an inhibitor of RdRp, targeting the viral genome replication process. Once the host has metabolised Remdesivir into the active metabolite, the latter competes with adenosine triphosphate (ATP; the natural nucleotide normally used in this process) for incorporation into the newly synthesised strand of RNA. Incorporation of this substitute into the new strand results in premature termination of RNA synthesis, when integrated at a specific point in the RNA chain, Remdesivir causes inhibition of RNA synthesis 5 nucleotides from the drug incorporation site, delaying chain termination and stopping RNA synthesis prematurely, stopping RNA strand growth after the addition of a few extra nucleotides. [61]

- Indication:

Covid-19 disease in adults and adolescents (>12 years and >40kg) with pneumonia requiring oxygen therapy. [52]

B. Lopinavir and Ritonavir

- Gross formula: C74H96N10O10S2 [62]
- IUPAC nomenclature:(2S)-N-[(2S ,4S ,5S)-5-[[2-(2,6-) dimethylphenoxy) acetyl]amino]-4-hydroxy-1,6-diphenylhexan-2-yl]-3-methyl-2-(2-oxo-1,3-diazinan-1- yl)butanamide;1,3-thiazol-5-ylmethyl N-[(2 S,3 S,5 S)-3-hydroxy-5-[[(2 S)-3methyl-2-[[methyl-[(2-propan-2-yl-1,3-thiazol-4 yl)methyl]carbamoyl]amino]butanoyl] amino]-1,6- diphenylhexan-2-yl]carbamate. [62]

- Mode of action

It is an antiretroviral active against the human immunodeficiency virus (HIV). The active ingredient is lopinavir, which belongs to the family of HIV protease inhibitors (antiproteases). By blocking this enzyme, it prevents the virus from reproducing in infected cells, but does not allow it to be eliminated. The other component is ritonavir, which is also an antiprotease, but which is not used in this combination at an antiviral dose, but at a dose that increases the concentrations of lopinavir in the body by inhibiting cytochrome P450 (so-called "booster" effect). [63]

- Indication

In HIV infection, in combination with other antiretroviral agents, including HIV reverse transcriptase inhibitors, in adult and pediatric patients over 14 days of age with progressive immune deficiency. [52]

In vitro and in vivo data, as well as clinical data in humans in the context of SARS-CoV and MERS-CoV coronavirus infections, have shown that the lopinavir/ritonavir combination has activity against these viruses. On this basis, in January 2020 the WHO recommended its evaluation in Covid- 19 disease at the same dose as in HIV infection; the results of these trials show that lopinavir/ritonavir alone or in combination with interferon beta were discontinued due to inefficacy. [64]

C. Paxlovid

The combination nirmatrelvir/ritonavir (Paxlovid, Pfizer laboratory), the first direct-acting antiviral, is active *per os*, within the framework of early access authorisation by the HAS for early curative treatment of pauci-symptomatic patients at high risk of severe Covid-19 disease. [65]

• Mode of action

Paxlovid® is an antiviral which prevents viral replication. It is a combination of nirmatrelvir and ritonavir, nirmatrelvir being an inhibitor of a cysteine residue responsible for the activity of the 3C-Like protease (3CL^{PRO}) of Sars-CoV- 2 [66].

3CLPRO is involved in the post-translational modification of a Sars-CoV-2 polyprotein, producing 16 non-structural proteins which play an essential role in viral replication, transcription and recombination during infection. Peptidase inhibition blocks the release of these non-structural proteins and limits the ineffectiveness of Sars-CoV-2. [67]

Ritonavir is a potent inhibitor of Cytochrome P450, which increases the blood concentration of Nirmatrelvir and prolongs its half-life, allowing it to be administered less frequently.

• Indication

Paxlovid® is indicated for the treatment of Covid-19 in adult patients who do not require oxygen therapy and who are at high risk of progression to a severe form of Covid-19 [68] for adults and children aged over 12 years or weighing more than 40kg. This drug was granted conditional marketing authorisation by the European Commission on 27 January 2022. [66]

^.1.4. Immunomodulators

A. Corticotherapy

The prescription of corticoids is discussed in the inflammatory phase of Covid-19 disease, in order to regulate the "cytokine storm". Clinically, this would correspond to a situation where the general symptoms persist, with patients being oxygen-reactive and having a biological inflammatory syndrome [64]. This was the first treatment to show a benefit on mortality in patients requiring oxygen therapy [69]. They can be administered orally or intravenously. [70]

❖ Dexamethasone and other glucocorticoids

• Gross formula: C22H29FO5 [53]

• IUPAC nomenclature: (8S,9R,10S,11S,13S,14S,16R,17R)-9-Fluoro-...
11,17-dihydroxy-17-(2-hydroxyacetyl)-10,13,16-trimethyl-
6,7,8,11,12,14,15,16 octahydrocyclopenta[a]phenanthren-3-one. [53]

- Chemical structure

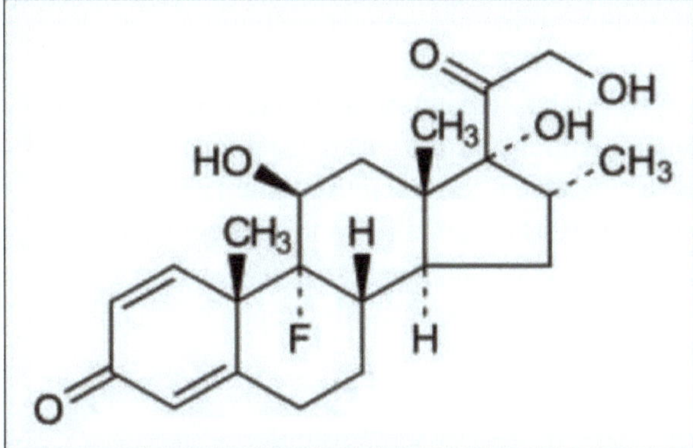

Figure 17: chemical structure of Dexamethasone. [53]

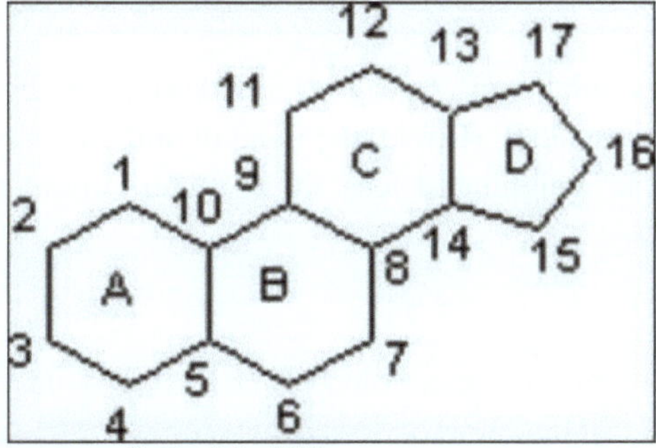

Figure 18: chemical structure of stdroi'de. [71]

- Relationship between chemical structure and therapeutic activity

All corticoids have a pregnane nucleus with common chemical groups that are essential for biological activity, but any modification can lead to a loss or increase in activity.

Cycle A :

The cetone function in position 3 and the unsaturation in 4-5 are essential for glucocorticoid activity. Unsaturation at 1-2 increases anti-inflammatory activity, while its elimination significantly increases mineralocorticoid activity. The addition of a pyrazole ring increases anti-inflammatory activity.

Cycle B :

Methylation at 6 promotes anti-inflammatory properties and reduces mineralocorticoid activity. Fluorination at C6 and C9 increases anti-inflammatory action and practically abolishes mineralocorticoid activity, and the same applies to unsaturation at 6-7.

Cycle C :

The OH group in 11P is essential for anti-inflammatory activity, while the cetone function promotes mineralocorticoid activity.

Cycle D :

Methylation in C16 (alpha or beta) or hydroxylation remarkably increases the anti-inflammatory potential and decreases the mineralocorticoid activity. The OH group at C17a is essential for the anti-inflammatory action of all corticoids. The cetone function at 20 is essential for glucocorticoid activity.

- Mode of action

Dexamethasone is mainly used as an anti-inflammatory agent.

Or immunosuppressant.

Their proposed mechanism in Sars-CoV-2 is the attenuation of an excessive immune response that can lead to acute respiratory distress syndrome⁖ (ARDS) and multi-organ failure. [72]

- Indication

Dexamethasone has obtained European marketing authorisation for the treatment of coronavirus 2019 (Covid-19) in adult and adolescent patients (aged 12 years and over and weighing at least 40 kg) who require additional oxygen therapy. [73]

B. Anakinra

- Mode of action

Anakinra is an antagonist of interleukin-1a (IL-1a) and interleukin-ip (IL-1p) receptors, major pro-inflammatory cytokines involved in the mediation of many cellular responses. [72] - Indication

Anakinra has marketing authorisation for the treatment of coronavirus 2019 (Covid-19) in adult patients with pneumonia requiring oxygen supplementation (low or high flow oxygen) and at risk of progressing to severe respiratory failure as evidenced by a plasma concentration of soluble urokinase-type plasminogen activator receptors (suPAR) > 6 ng/mL. [59]

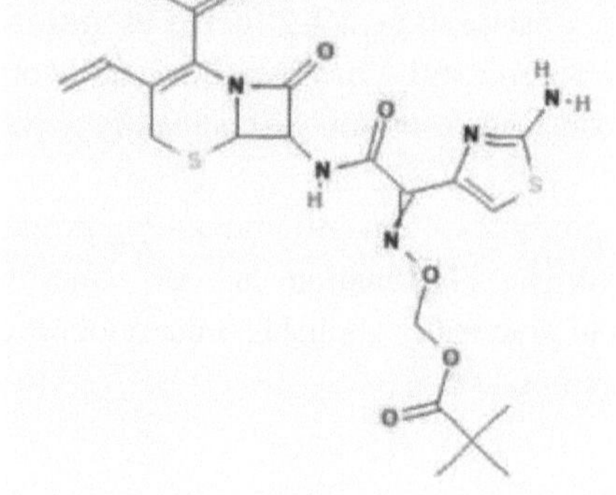

Figure 19: chemical structure of Anakinra. [74]

C. Tocilizumab

- Mode of action

It is a humanised IgG1 monoclonal antibody directed against the soluble and membrane receptor for human mterleukme-6 (IL-6), thus inhibiting the pro-inflammatory properties of IL-6. [52]

- Indication

Roactemra (Tocilizumab) has a specific marketing authorisation for the treatment of Covid-19 in adults receiving systemic corticotherapie and oxygen-requiring or requiring mechanical ventilation and having a marked inflammatory state (CRP > 75 mg/L). [59]

The HCSP does not recommend the use of Tocilizumab in patients undergoing invasive mechanical ventilation. [59]

^.1.5. Post-exposure prophylaxis

It is indicated for adult patients and children aged 12 and over who are immunocompromised and unprotected despite a full vaccination schedule. [75]

A. Bamlanivimab ± Etesivimab :

In France, the ANSM has granted a cohort ATU (starting date 22/02/2021 and closing date 31 December 2021) for the use of Bamlanivimab in the treatment of mild to moderate symptomatic forms of Covid-19 in adults with a positive virological test for Sars-CoV-2 and at high risk of progression to a severe form of the disease. [76] - Mode of action :

These 2 anti-spike neutralising monoclonal antibodies come from 2 separate patients who recovered from Covid-19 in North America and China respectively.

Bamlanivimab is an IgG1 neutralising monoclonal antibody directed against the viral spike protein, designed to block viral anchorage and entry into human cells.

Etesevimab is a neutralising monoclonal antibody directed against the Sars-CoV-2 surface protein, protein S (or Spike protein). In preclinical studies, it has been shown that Etesevimab binds to a different epitope from Bamlanivimab and neutralises Bamlanivimab-resistant mutants, which justifies the interest of combining these two antibodies in patients with Covid-19 [72].

B. Casirivimab and Imdevimab

Casirivimab and lmdevimab are monoclonal antibodies specifically directed against the surface protein of Sars-CoV-2, protein S, designed to block the attachment and entry of the virus into human cells. [72]

The combination of Casirivimab and Imdevimab is indicated for post-exposure prophylaxis of Sars-CoV-2 infection in adults and children aged >12 years and weighing >40 kg at high risk of progression to a severe form of the disease, who are unvaccinated or have a medical condition (pathology or treatment) making a response to vaccine protection unlikely. [77]

A. Analgesics and antipyretics

❖ Paracetamol (Acetaminophen)

- Gross formula C8H9NO2 [53]
- IUPAC nomenclature: N-(4-Hydroxyphenyl) acetamide [53].
- Chemical structure :

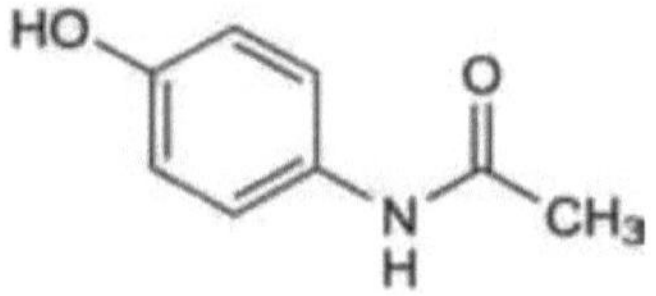

Figure 20: chemical structure of Paracetamol. [53]

- Mode of action

Paracetamol acts on the central nervous system (CNS), is highly lipophilic and penetrates the brain very rapidly. [78] Cyclooxygenases (COX) are part of an enzyme complex that converts arachidonic acid into prostaglandin H2 (PGH2) [79]. In the presence of peroxide groups (H_2O_2). The free phenol function of paracetamol captures peroxide groups from the environment, thus inhibiting the peroxidase function of the cerebral-specific COX-2.

One hypothesis of a preferential action on a specific COX-3 of the central nervous system is invalid because this protein, although found in humans, lacks COX-type properties. [80] Another hypothesis explains that it exerts analgesic effects in the CNS by potentiating serotonin neurons descending from the spinal cord, which has the effect of exerting inhibitory control over nociceptive pathways. [79]

- Indication: Paracetamol is an antipyretic analgesic with no anti-inflammatory activity [78]. It is indicated for the symptomatic treatment of painful and/or febrile conditions. [52]

Why are non-steroidal anti-inflammatory drugs (NSAIDs) not recommended in the treatment of Covid-19?

Non-steroidal anti-inflammatories are not recommended. Paracetamol is recommended to treat headaches and aches, or to reduce fever. [81]

NSAIDs are thought to increase the risk of bacterial infections, pleuropulmonary complications (empyema), dissemination of infection, prolongation of the disease in children and adults, and the risk of aggravating Covid-19 susceptibility factors (such as a cardiovascular accident or deterioration in renal function). [82]

B. Anticoagulants :

A large proportion of patients with Covid-19 develop coagulation disorders of varying degrees of severity, secondary to infection with Sars-CoV-2. This high thrombotic risk is thought to be the result of excessive systemic inflammation due to an uncontrolled immune response. Prolonged immobilisation and the presence of conventional cardiovascular risk factors also contribute to the thromboembolic risk. [83] - Indication

This is why the use of anticoagulants (low molecular weight heparin or Fondaparinux) is recommended. As prophylaxis for non-oxygen-dependent subjects, whether hospitalised or not, and presenting risk factors for venous thromboembolism (VTE). [84]

I V.2. Medical supplements

^.2.1. Vitamins

A. Vitamin D

It has a structure similar to that of cholesterol (Figure 21), and is a fat-soluble vitamin synthesised in the human body from a cholesterol derivative under the action of UVB radiation from light. It exists in two forms: D2 (ergocalciferol) or D3 (cholecalciferol). [85]

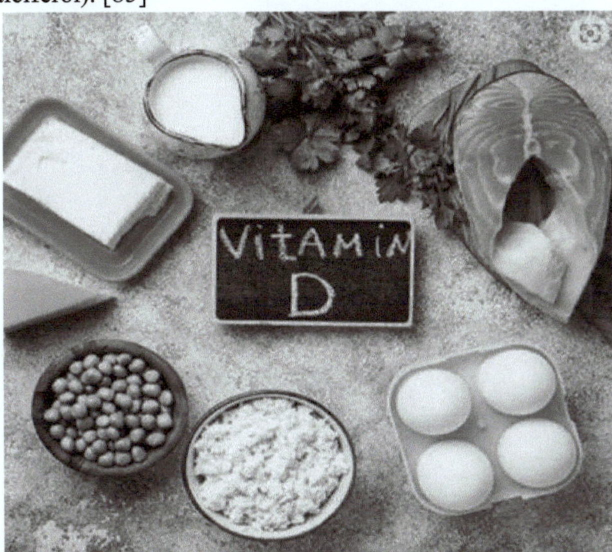

Figure 21: dietary sources of Vitamin D. [85]

Vitamin D3 is a pro-hormone known for its key role in calcium metabolism (intestinal absorption, bone binding). But it has other unconventional effects. In particular, it modulates immune system function by stimulating macrophages and dendritic cells. It plays a role in regulating and suppressing the inflammatory cytokine response that causes respiratory distress syndrome ждиё [86], Vitamin D supplementation could done reduce the risk of occurrence and severity of infection in Covid-19 disease. [87]

B. Ascorbic acid (Vitamin C)

Vitamin C is a powerful antioxidant, an effective scavenger of reactive oxygen and nitrogen species. It is used in the treatment of Covid-19 by improving the innate antimicrobial immune response and reducing unnecessary inflammatory reactions, thereby minimising the risk of inflammation-related cell damage. A high dose reduces the risk of a cytokine storm by reducing pro-inflammatory cytokine levels in the blood. [89]

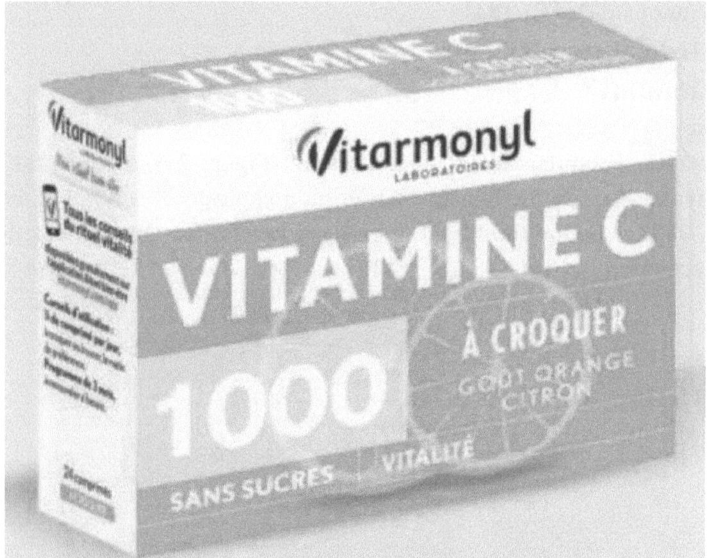

Figure 22: Ascorbic acid (vitamin C) in commercial medicinal form. [88]

IV.2.2. Oligoelements

❖ Le Zinc

Zinc is best known for its action on the skin, nails and hair, and is a powerful antioxidant (like selenium and vitamin C) because it can prevent the production of free radicals. But zinc can improve the function of the immune system by: increasing the activity of T-helper 1 cells, which are mainly anti-inflammatory; and suppressing the function of effector T cells, which are mainly pro-inflammatory. It also has an effect on cognitive function and plays a role in protein synthesis and the maintenance of normal vision. [90]

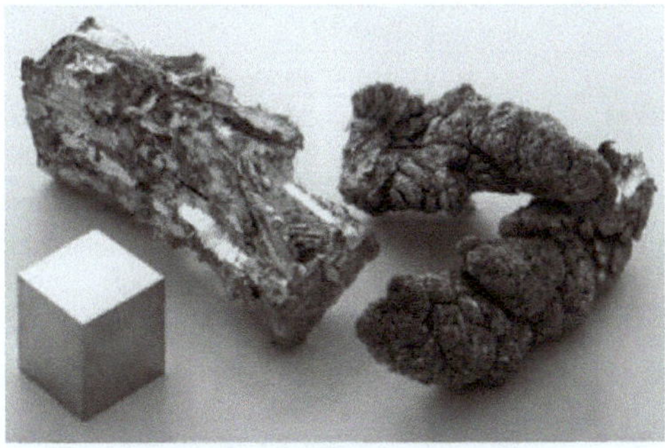

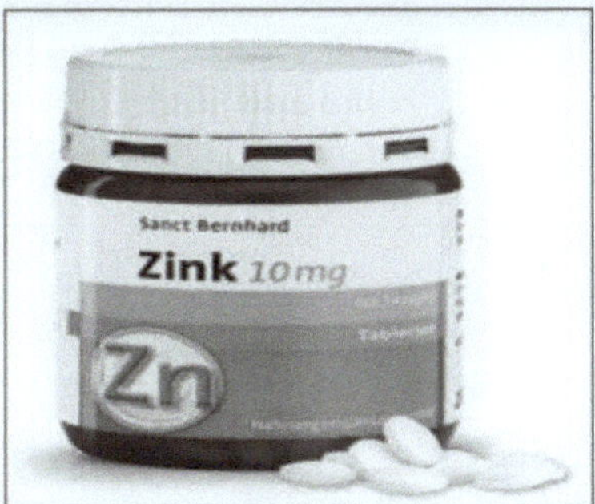

Figure 23: **(A)** 99.99% pure crystalline zinc vs **(B)** compressed pharmaceutical zinc.

IV.3. Vaccines against Covid-19

The principle behind vaccines is to enable the immune system to trigger a specific immune response against Sars-CoV-2 and neutralise it before it has time to develop Covid-19 disease (or mitigate its consequences). Most vaccines target the virus's spike protein (S protein).

Different vaccine technologies are used to vaccinate against Covid-19:

- Traditional technologies, based on the use of a whole, inactive virus, in this case Sars-CoV-2, or the use of just one part of the virus (usually a protein, in this case the S protein) (e.g. Novavax vaccines), combined with an immune adjuvant.

-New technologies, based on :

- The use of "pure" nucleic acid (DNA or RNA), i.e. the gene sequence of the target protein: in this case protein S.
- Using a viral vector in which the gene for the target protein has been inserted, the Sars-CoV-2 protein. [91]
-

Table 2: Covid-19 vaccines worldwide (2023 data) [92].

Names of vaccines	Type of vaccine
Spoutnik V® (Gamaleya)	Anti-Covid 19 vaccine with a non-replicating viral vector (Adenovirus).
Comirnaty®(PfizerBioNTech)	Nucleoside-modified messenger RNA vaccine against Covid-19.
Spikevax® (Moderna)	Anti-Covid 19 vaccine has mRNA.
Vaxzevria® (Astrazeneca)	Anti-Covid 19 vaccine with a non-replicating viral vector (chimpanzee adenovirus).
JCOVDEN® (Janssen)	Non-replicating viral vector vaccine (Adenovirus).
NUVAXOVID® (Novavax)	Recombinant nanoparticle subunit vaccine with adjuvant (Matrix M).
CoronaVac® (Sinovac)	Inactivated adjuvanted Sars-CoV-2 vaccine (a substance which helps to strengthen the immune system ace vaccine).
COVILO® (Sinopharm)	Inactive whole Sars-CoV-2 vaccine.
COVAXIN® (Bharat biotech)	Inactive whole vaccine against Covid-19 adjuvanted with a molecule from the class of imidazoquinoline agonists of TLR 7 and 8 adsorbed onto aluminium hydroxide.

Chapter V

Algerian plants with anti-Covid-19 potential

V .1. White wormwood or *Artemisia herba alba*

V .1.1. Biological and pharmacological properties

It is used to treat gastric and hepatic disorders, as well as a wide range of other ailments, and against certain forms of poisoning. It is also used to treat diabetes, bronchitis, abscess, diarrhoea and as a vermifuge. It has obvious purgative properties playing a great role in the control of intestinal worms. [93]

One review mentions its antioxidant, anti-venom, antifungal, nematocidal, antibacterial, antispasmodic, anthelmintic, anti-leishmanial, neurological (Alzheimer's disease, epilepsy and depression) and hypoglycemic properties.

In Silico, phytochemical compounds from Artemisia herba-alba have a high probability of binding to Sars-CoV-2 Mpro, inhibiting protease with consequent blockage of viral replication. [94]

V .1.2. Chemical composition :

- Terpenes of Artemisia herba-alba :

Terpenes are polymers made up of C5 units. Monoterpenes (C10) are slightly volatile substances that form essential oils. They protect plants from parasites, inhibit bacterial growth and attract pollinating animals.

The main monoterpenes identified in *Artemisia herba alba* are: thujone (monoterpenelactone), 1,8-cineol and thymol.

Thujone is one of the most bioactive terpenic constituents of wormwood. Structurally related to menthol, it consists of a C6 ring (cyclohexane) plus an exocyclic isopropyl group and a lactone group. Hujone is a chiral compound present in its natural state in the form of two stereoisomers: talpha-thujone and beta- thujone. [95]

A/

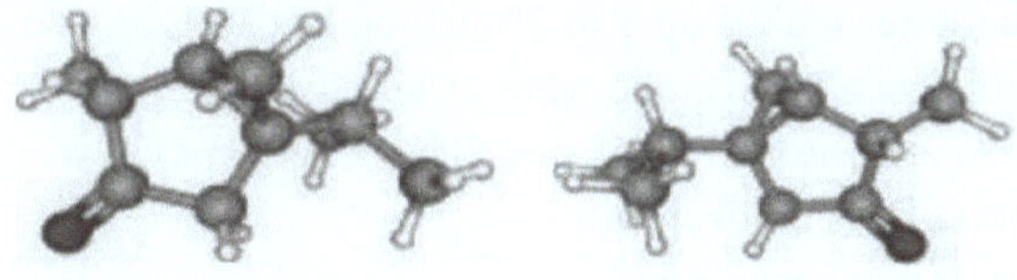

B/

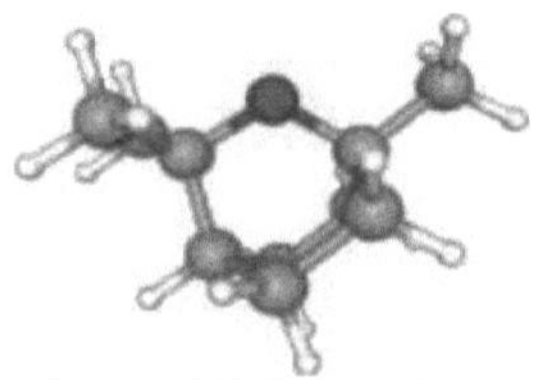

Figure 24: A/ 3D structure of a-thujone and P-thujone (C10H10O) [96].
B/ 3D structure of 1,8-cineol-d3 (C10H18O) [97].

- Flavonoides of Artemisia herba-alba :
The main flavonoids are hispidulin (4',5,7-trihydroxy-6- methoxyflavone) and 12-cirsimaritine. [95]

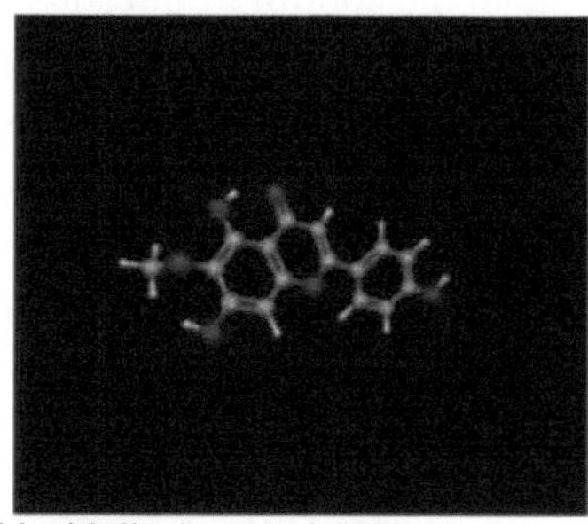

Figure 25: 3D structure of 1 hispidulin (C16H12O6) [98].

V.1.4 Indication in phytotherapy
-Part used: leaves and flowering tops.
-Forms of use: gelules, powders, dried leaves, essential oil.
-Internal use: Herbal tea to treat bronchitis, coughs, diabetes, high blood pressure and diarrhoea.
-External use: The essential oil of 1 armoise is used in friction or massage against rheumatism and painful parts of the body. [99]

V .2. Laurier noble or *Laurus nobilis L*

V .2.1. Chemical composition of the plant

The leaves of *Laurus nobilis* contain several active substances, including essential oils. The latter makes up 1 to 3% of the dry weight, and contains 30 to 70% of 1-8 cineol (eucalyptol), and several terpenic compounds: linalool (8 to 16%), eugenol 3%, pinene and terpinene. The leaves may also contain tannins and polar and apolar flavonoids. [100]

V .2.2. Pharmacological properties

-All three extracts (essential oil, ethanolic extract and decoction) have antioxidant activity. [101]

-Cytotoxic effect: Certain compounds isolated from *Laurus nobilis L* have been shown to be cytotoxic, essentially the two sesquiterpenes; lactones and lauroxe.

These active substances are highly cytotoxic against the cancerous ovarian cell line. [102]

Antimicrobial effect: antimicrobial activity of *L.nobilis* essential oil against the Gram-positive bacterial (*S.aureus*) and BGN (*E.coli* and *P.aeruginosa*) strains tested, as well as against the fungus *C. albicans*. The highest activity was observed in *S. aureus*. [103]

-   Laurel essential oil is also a powerful virucide. The combination of 1,8-cineole and monoterpenols is very effective in treating viral lower ENT pathologies (coronarovirus, SARS-coV, Herpes virus [HSV-1]). [104]

-   Noble Laurel EO is also capable of stimulating immunity. In experiments, 1,8-cineole demonstrated its immunostimulant properties by increasing y-globulins and P-globulins. [104]

-   Gastro-protective effect: the decoction and methanolic extracts have an effect on stomach protection against ulcerations and stimulate appetite. [102]

-   .2.3 Indication in phytotherapy

•   Parts used: Leaves and fruit (berries).

•   Uses: as a decoction or herbal tea of noble laurel. Alternatively ;

Laurel butter or oil: extracted from desiccated fruit, pulverised and exposed to boiling water.

-Internal use: For digestive disorders and insufficient perspiration in the form of infusion.

- External use: Joint and rheumatic pain. [105]

V.3. Nigella or *Nigella sativa L*

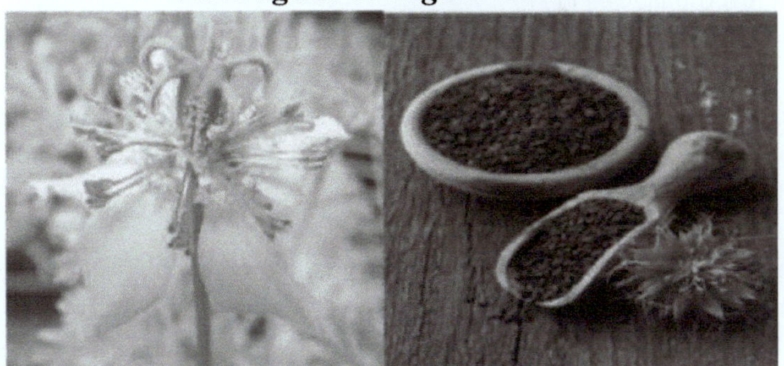

Figure 26: *Nigella sativa* flowers and seeds [106].

V.3.1. Chemical composition of the plant

The active constituents of *N.sativa* are thymohydroquinone, p-cymene, dithymoquinone, thymoquinone, carvacrol and sesquiterpene longifolene. *N. sativa* seeds also contain pentacyclic triterpene, alpha-hederin, proteins, carbohydrates, crude fibre, lipids and saponin. N. sativa oil contains oleic acid, palmitic acid and linoleic acid. Aromatic compounds contain a-thuyene, thymol,

39

a-pinene, thymoquinone, dihydrothymoquinone. [107]

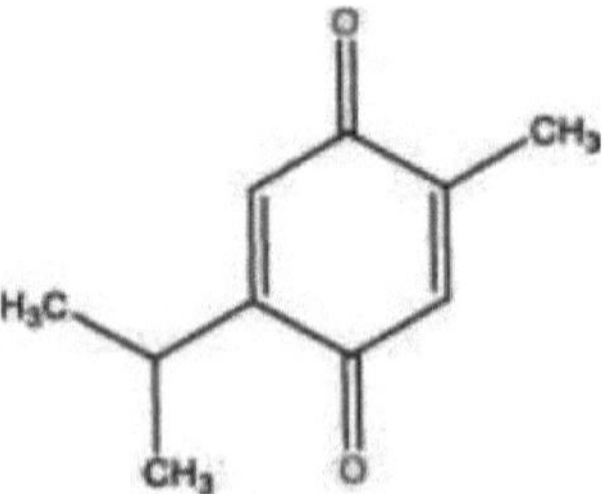

Figure 27: Chemical structure of Thymoquinone. [108]

V .3.2. Pharmacological properties

-Anti-inflammatory activity: it has an anti-inflammatory activity which has proved particularly effective against certain inflammatory diseases such as colitis, peritonitis, arthritis and asthma. [109]

-Antimicrobial action: Black cumin is often presented as a natural anti-infective, with antibacterial, antiparasitic, antiviral and antifungal action. [110]

-Antispasmodic effect: it also appears to have an antispasmodic effect, preventing the onset of spasms in the respiratory tract, muscular spasms, gastric spasms, intestinal spasms and uterine spasms... [107]

-Immunostimulant effect: in vitro, it has immunopotentiating properties for T lymphocytes. In fact, seed extracts activate the secretion of Interleukin-3 (IL-3) and increase the production of IL-ip by T lymphocytes, indicating a stimulatory effect on macrophages. [111]

Black cumin also has gastro-protective, anti-cancer, emmenagogue and anti-diabetic properties. [112]

In silico studies show that four phytochemicals from *N. sativa,* a-hederine, dithymoquinone, neglacin and negerillidin, have the potential to inhibit the RdRp of Sars-CoV-2. [113]

V .3.3. Form of use

The essential oil is the most widely used form, and there are also gelules, herbal teas and Nigella soap.

Internal use: The oil in the bottle is recommended for both internal and external use. The recommended dosage for the capsules is 2 to 4 capsules at 500 mg per day in the middle of a meal for an adult and 1 to 2 capsules per day for a child.

External use in phytotherapy: black cumin oil is generally used pure, applied locally several times a day; it can also be added to boiling water before being inhaled. [114]

V .4. Eucalyptus or *Eucalyptus globulus*

V .4.1. Chemical composition of the plant

The leaves of the common eucalyptus contain 1 to 3% essential oil.*Eucalyptus globulus* EO has the following composition:

* Terpene oxides: 1,8 cineole (eucalyptol).
* Monoterpenes: alpha-pinene, limonene, gamma-terpinene, paracymene.
* Sesquiterpenes: aromadendrene.
* Sesquiterpenes: globulol, ledol.
* Flavonoids: Flavone heterosides with the following aglycones: quercetin, myricetin, k^mpferol and rutin. [115]

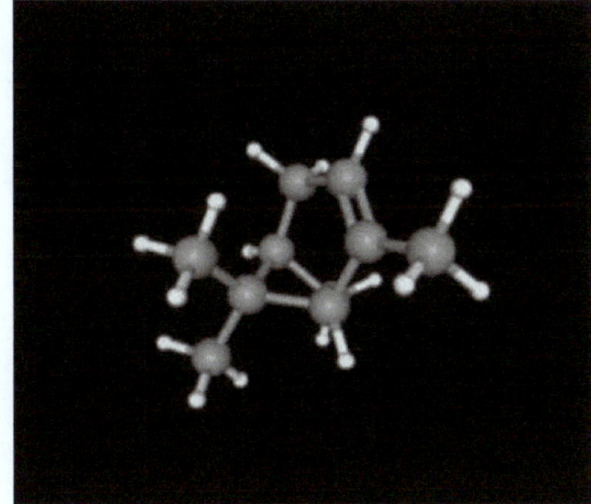

Figure 28: 3D structure of alpha-pinene ($C_{10}H_{16}$) [116].

V .4.2. Pharmacological properties

The WHO recognises the traditional use of Eucalyptus leaves as a urinary tract antiseptic, analgesic for internal and external use, antihistamine, antiviral, antitumour, antifungal and antimalarial. They are also used in the prevention and treatment of cardiovascular disease, hypoglycaemic and bronchial antispasmodics and to relieve fever and asthma symptoms. [117]

Eucalyptus globulus essential oil is used as an antiseptic and antispasmodic agent in bronchitis, asthma and minor respiratory ailments. They have cough suppressant, expectorant and mucolytic properties. [117]

Several studies have shown antimicrobial activity against both Gram-negative and Gram-positive bacteria. [117]

V .4.3 Indication in phytotherapy

Parts used: Leaves and wood.

Forms of use: Hydrolate (refrigerated storage, maximum 6 months after opening), nebulisate, fluid extract, infusion, tincture, balms and ointments.

Internal use: bronchial infections

External use: infusion or bath: 3 litres of infusion in the bath. This method

takes advantage of the balsamic and antiseptic benefits of eucalyptus leaves.
[118]

V .5. Cloves: *Syzygium aromaticum*

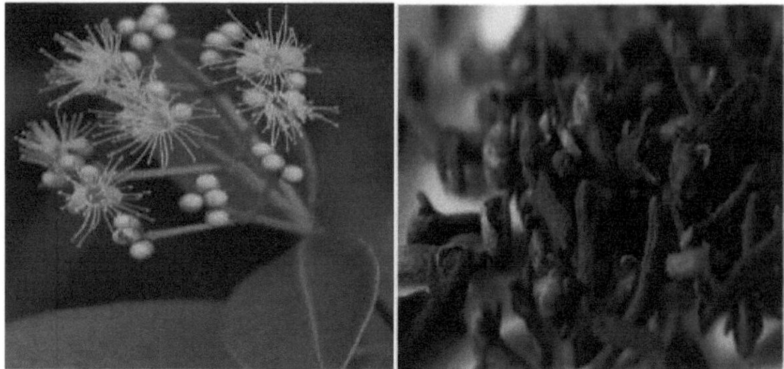

Figure 29: *Syzyguim aramaticum* [119]

V .5.1. Chemical composition of the plant :
Cloves are rich in bioactive substances, containing 15% essential oil composed
of 70-90% eugenol, an antibacterial, antiseptic and antifungal substance. It also
contains between 9 and 15% eugenol acetate, between 5 and 12% alpha- and
beta- caryophyllene, 2% oleanic acid and methyl salicylate [120]. It also
contains gums and tannins [121].

V .5.2. Pharmacological properties :
-*Analgesics*: It is used for all types of mouth pain. It contributes to the
suppression of bacteria, which cause the development of bad breath. [123]

V *Gastro-protective activity:* Cloves have digestive properties. It improves
digestive comfort and helps restore the intestinal microbiota. [123]

V *Anti-inflammatory properties:* It helps to treat inflammation.
In fact, the antioxidants in cloves are highly active.
[123]

V *Immunomodulating activity:* It should be noted that clove is a powerful
antiviral, helping to fight viral infections while stimulating immunity. [123]

V *Antiseptic*: they are effective in the treatment of certain viral diseases in
tropical Asia: in cases of malaria, cholera and tuberculosis, or parasites such as
scabies. [121]

V .5.3 Indication in phytotherapy
- *Forms of use:*
As an infusion of cloves and tincture for the treatment of flatulence and essential
oils in the treatment of dental pain. cloves can cause skin reactions when used
externally. [121] - *Parts used*: the flower buds are used as infusions or powders

and essential oils are extracted. The leaves and stems are sometimes used to extract the essential oil. [121]

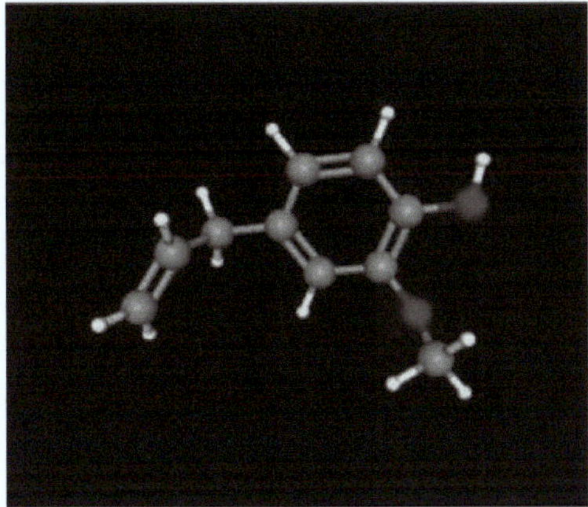

Figure 30: 3D structure of eugdnol ($C_{10}H_{12}O_2$) [122].

Chapter VI

The after-effects of Covid-19

VI.1 Definition

Post-Covid sequelae, also known as "Covid long" or "post-Covid syndrome", are defined as signs and symptoms developed during or after an acute Sars-CoV-2 infection. They persist for more than four weeks, are not explained by other diagnoses and have an impact on daily life. [124]

Table 3: WHO definition of protracted forms of Covid-19 [125].

WHO definition of prolonged forms of Covid-19
- Persistence or recurrence of symptoms
- Within 12 weeks of a Covid-19 episode and generally lasting more than 2 months
- Confirmed or highly probable (according to HAS definition)
- Occurring during epidemics
- With no other explanation for the onset of these symptoms

VI.2 Delay of post-Covid symptoms

The NICE guideline proposes the following classification: Covid-19 acuteC (symptoms up to 4 weeks), Covid symptomatic continuous (symptoms from 4 to 12 weeks) and post Covid (symptoms appearing during or after an infection and persisting for more than 12 weeks). In this guideline, the term "long Covid" would include the two subgroups, continuous symptomatic Covid and post-Covid syndrome [124]. In a subsequent review of the NICE guideline, Sivan and Taylor proposed the unified definition of long Covid as "signs and symptoms that persist for more than four weeks and can be attributed to Covid-19 infection".

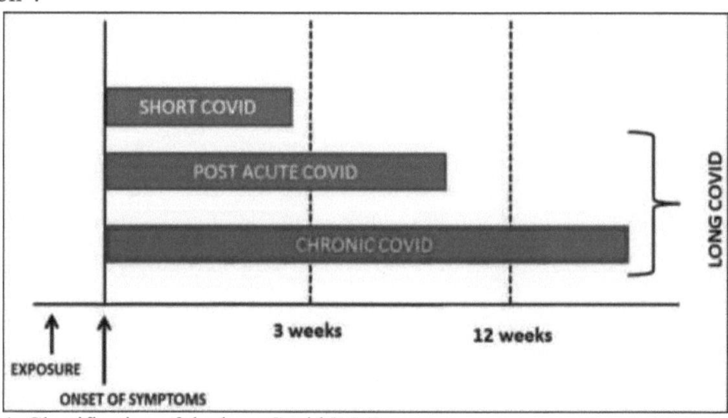

Figure 31: Classification of the long Covid [126].

We are talking about post-Covid sequelae, which often affect patients who have experienced severe or critical forms of the disease. For example, pulmonary fibrosis may result from respiratory distress, chronic renal damage may result from ждиё renal failure, and cardiac lesions (myocarditis, ventricular failure, myocardial infarction, etc...) may be secondary to the inflammation and hemodynamic complications that occurred during the infection. These sequelae may be reversible or definitive. [37]

Certain symptoms of Covid-19 may persist for several weeks, or even months, even though the virus is no longer detectable in the patient's body and the patient has not developed a severe form of the disease. These prolonged symptoms are most often: chronic fatigue, neurocognitive disorders, digestive disorders, cardiopulmonary signs (dyspnea, chest pain and/or tightness, cough, tachycardia) or musculoskeletal pain. They form what is known as **Covid long**. These signs evolve in a fluctuating manner, but tend towards a slowly progressive improvement. [37]

In addition, the disease has an impact on mental health, with a risk of developing anxiety or depression among patients and their relatives, as well as among the carers who have looked after the patients. Post-traumatic stress disorders have also been reported in people admitted to intensive care units, as well as their carers. [37]

VI.3 Survey in Algeria 2023

VI.3.1. Materials and Methods

A. Study framework

From an epidemiological point of view, this is a retrospective descriptive study. This study consists of a survey carried out using an anonymous, simple and rapid questionnaire distributed in hybrid mode in two formats: online (with GoogleForm®) and on a printed form to be distributed in face-to-face mode to the Algerian population in French.

B. Description of the zone

Algeria is a country in North Africa, bordered by the Mediterranean Sea, Tunisia to the north-east, Libya to the east, Niger to the south-east, Mali, Mauritania and the Western Sahara to the south-west, and Morocco to the west. It is regarded as a bridge between Africa and Europe.

Algeria covers an area of 2,381,741 km^2 , making it the largest country in Africa and the tenth largest in the world. Situated in the north-west of the African continent, with a coastline on the Mediterranean Sea that is home to almost the entire population and a desert interior that makes up 85% of the entire territory.

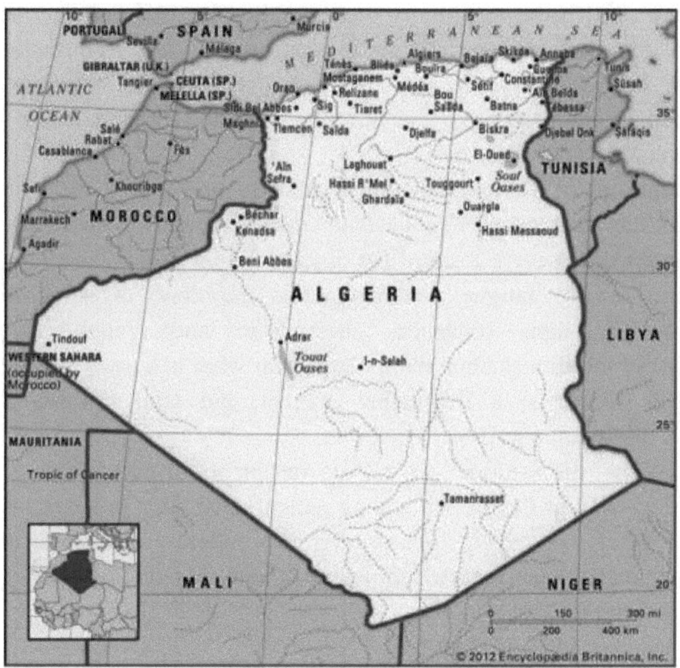

Figure 32: Graphical map of Algoie. [127]

The target population

It has been estimated that the population of Algeria will be 46,116,000 in 2023 [127], and its density is very unevenly distributed, with most people living on the northern coasts of the country. The target population for this study is only people living in Algeria, given that the questionnaire is online and distributed face-to-face. At the end of the survey period, 335 participants responded to our questionnaire.

•   **Inclusion criteria**: We retrospectively included all patients aged from less than 18 years to more than 50 years, with or without comorbidities. We wanted our study to be wide-ranging and to reach all age groups and categories of the population.

•   **Non-inclusion criteria**: There were no non-inclusion or exclusion criteria.

C. Duration of study

The survey was carried out between 20 January 2023 and 20 April 2023.

D. Questionnaire used

Our study was carried out using a survey form in the form of a questionnaire based on 3 headings (Appendix 1)

•   The first section is designed to collect the socio-demographic characteristics

46

of the respondents: sex, wilaya of residence, age, social situation, intellectual level and the presence or absence of co-morbidity.

• The second section deals with the Sars-CoV-2 infection, the symptoms experienced by people suffering from the disease, the different tests and Covid's vaccine. As well as the type of treatment used (medical or phytotherapeutic).

• The third section deals with the organic and psychosocial sequelae of Sars-CoV-2, the symptoms of long covid and its impact on people's lives.

The questionnaire included questions with suggested answers, open questions, short answer questions and paragraph-type questions.

a. Data processing

All responses are automatically saved in a Google Forms spreadsheet in chronological order, and can be downloaded in Excel format. In order to better organise the work, the downloaded file was subsequently copied and modified in several tables on Microsoft Excel 2019, which enabled all the parameters to be examined, giving all the functions required for the study.

IV.3.2. Results

A. Descriptive parameters of the population

• *Breakdown of the population by gender*

Of the 335 respondents to the questionnaire, 72% were women and 28% were men. The diagrams below show the distribution of respondents by gender (Table 4 and Figure 33).

Table 4: Breakdown of people by gender.

Gender	Workforce	Percentage
Fdminin	241	72%
Male	94	28%
Total	335	100%

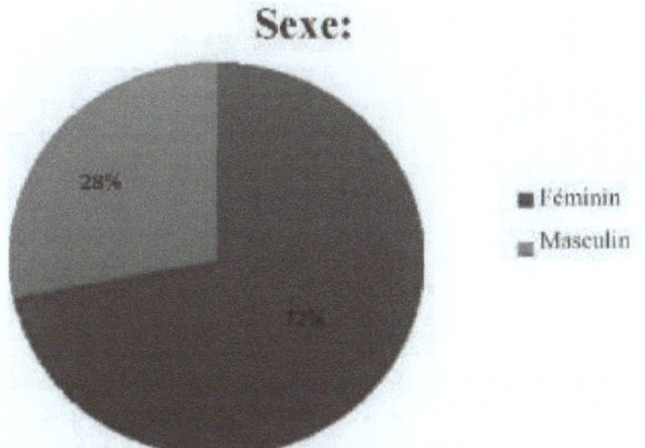

Figure 33: Breakdown of respondents by gender.

• *Breakdown of the population by age*

47

The age group that responded most to our study questionnaire was young people aged between 18 and 30 (208 patients or 62%), followed by people aged between 30 and 50 with a percentage of 23%. (Table 5, Figure 34)

Table 5: Breakdown of people by age.

Age group :	< 18	[18-30[	[30-50[	Over 50s	Total
Workforce	6	208	76	45	335
Percentage	2%	62%	23%	13%	100%

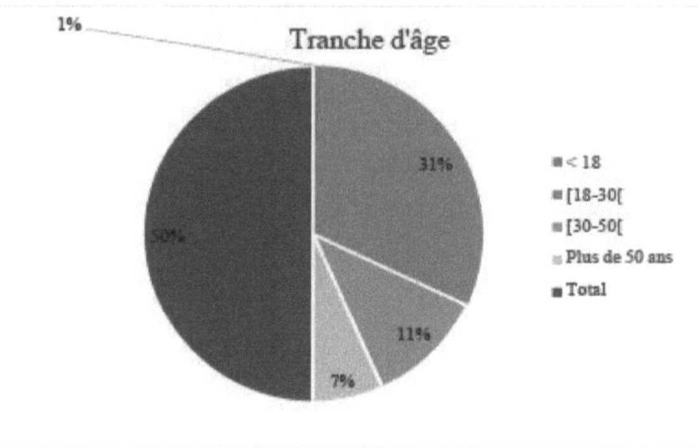

Figure 34: Rëpartition of people by age.

- Breakdown of the population by place of residence
Of the 335 patients, the inhabitants of El Taref and Annaba were the most likely to respond to the questionnaire, with percentages of 34% and 32% respectively. For the rest of the population, 8% of patients lived in the wilaya of Skikda and 4% in Algiers and Soug Ahrass (Table 6 and Figure 35).

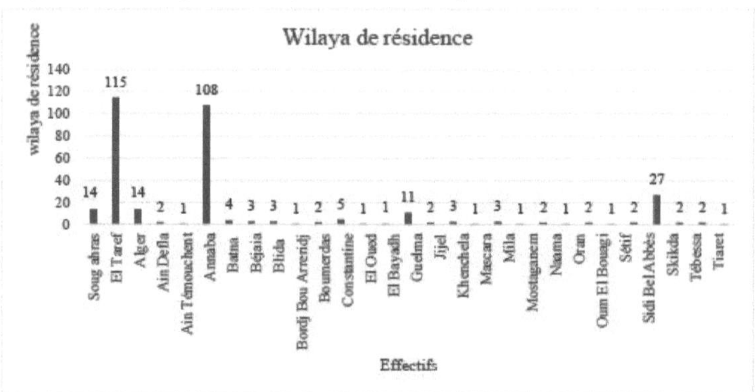

Figure 35: Rëpartition of the population by wilaya of residence.

Wilaya	Workforce	Percentage
Soug Ahras	14	4,18%
El Taref	115	34,33%
Algiers	14	4,18%

Ain Defla	2	0,60%
Ain Tëmouchent	1	0,30%
Annaba	108	32,24%
Batna	4	1,19%
Bejaia	3	0,90%
Blida	3	0,90%
Bordj Bou Arreridj	1	0,30%
Boumerdas	2	0,60%
Constantine	5	1,49%
El Oued	1	0,30%
El Bayadh	1	0,30%
Guelma	11	3,28%
Jijel	2	0,60%
Khenchela	3	0,90%
Mascara	1	0,30%
Mila	3	0,90%
Mostaganem	1	0,30%
Naama	2	0,60%
Oran	1	0,30%
Oum El Bouagi	2	0,60%
Sëtif	1	0,30%
Sidi Bel Abbës	2	0,60%
Skikda	27	8,06%
Tëbessa	2	0,60%
Tiaret	2	0,60%
Tlemcen	1	0,30%
Total	335	100%

Most of the subjects surveyed, 77% (257 people), had a higher level of education. Of the remaining subjects, 8% had a secondary level of education, 7% had not attended school and 6% had an intermediate level of education. (Table 7 figure 36)

Tableau 7:   Breakdown of the population by level of education.

Level of education	Workforce	Percentage
Medium	21	6%
Not at school	25	7%
Primary	6	2%
Secondary	26	8%
University	257	77%
Total	335	100%

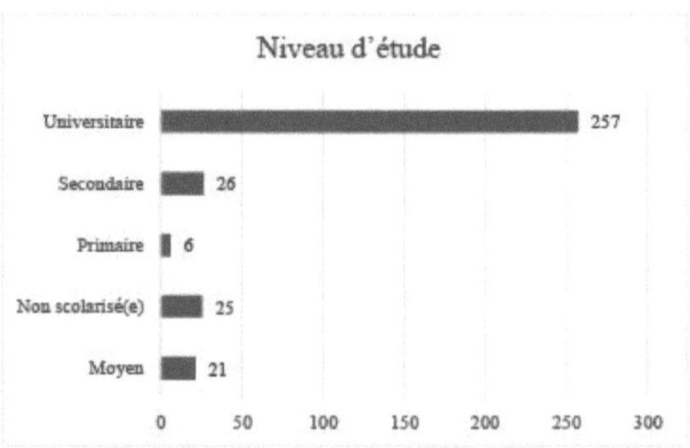

Figure 36: Breakdown of respondents by level of education.

- Breakdown of the population by social situation
More than half the population (65%, 217 people) are single, and 35% are married. (Table 8, Figure 37)

Tableau 8:   Breakdown of people by marital status.

Social situation	Single	Marie	Total
Workforce	217	118	335
Percentage	35%	65%	100 %

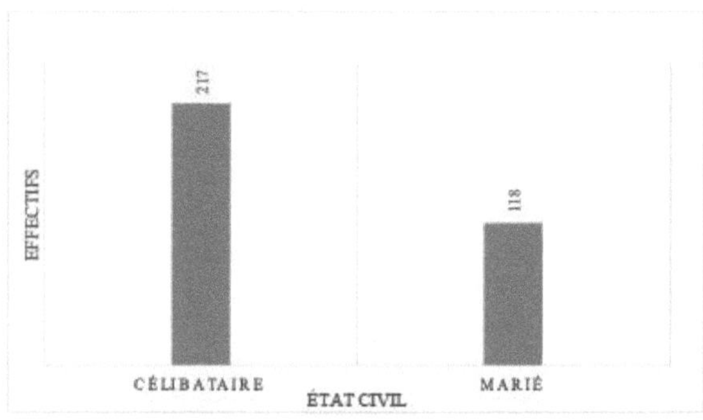

Figure 37: Breakdown of people by marital status.

- Breakdown of the population by socio-professional category
In terms of socio-professional category, half of the subjects surveyed, i.e. 50% (168), were students. Of the remaining subjects, 23% were civil servants and 16% were unemployed. (Table 9 and figure 38)

Tableau 9:   Breakdown of the population by socio-professional category.

Socio-professional category	Retailer	Student (e)	Functional	Withdrawal e	Unemployed	Total
Workforce	20	168	78	17	52	335
Percentage	6%	50%	23%	5%	16%	100%

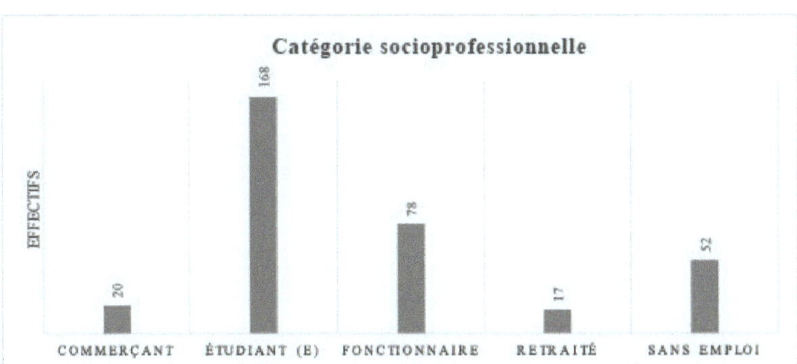

Figure 38: Breakdown of the population by socio-professional category.

Breakdown of the population according to the presence of a chronic illness
A total of 261 people (78%) of the subjects surveyed have no chronic disease, while 74 people (22%) are affected (Table 10 and figure 39); of which cardiovascular disease, respiratory disease and diabetes represent 26%, 20% and 22% of chronic diseases. (Table 11 and figure 40).

Tableau 10:   Frequency and percentage of people with or without a chronic disease.

Chronic illness	Workforce	Percentage
No	261	78%
Yes	74	22%
Total	335	100%

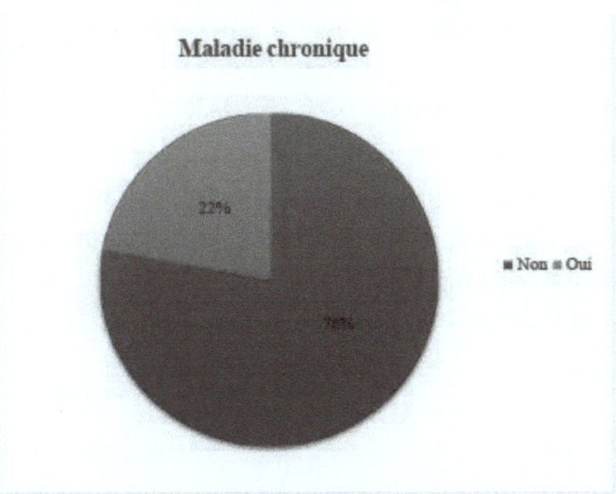

Figure 39: Frequency and percentage of people with or without a chronic illness.

Tableau 11:   Type of chronic disease present in the study population.

Chronic illness	Workforce	Percentage
Diabetes	23	21,70%

Cardiovascular disease	28	26,42%
Respiratory disease	21	19,81%
Celiac disease	7	6,60%
Thyroi'dite	11	10,38%
Renal failure	0	0,00%
Hëpatic insufficiency	0	0,00%
Rheumatoid arthritis	5	4,72%
Cancer	1	0,94%
Benign prostatic hypertrophy	2	1,89%
AVC	1	0,94%
Allergic rhinitis	1	0,94%
Glaucoma	1	0,94%
Coagulopathy	4	3,77%
Parkinson's disease	1	0,94%
Total	106	100%

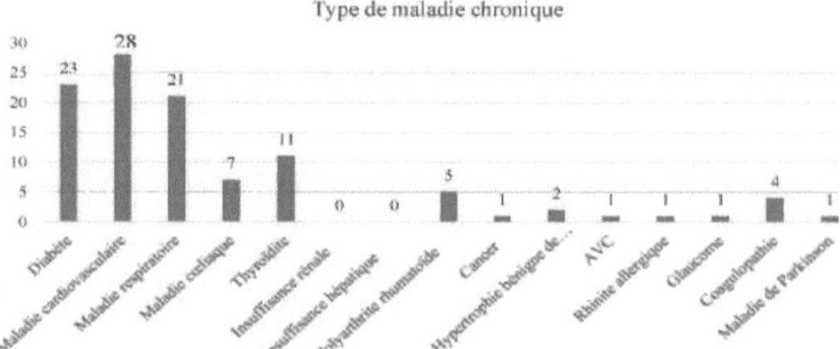

Figure 40: Type of chronic disease present in the study population.

B. Involvement and treatment of Covid-19

- Breakdown of the population by Covid-19 status

Almost all of the population surveyed caught up with Covid-19, with a percentage of 99%. The responses collected are organised in the tables and diagrams below Table 12 and figure 41.

Table 12: Breakdown of the population according to Covid-19 status.

Covid-19	Workforce	Percentage
No	5	1%
Yes	330	99%
Total	335	100,00%

Covid-19

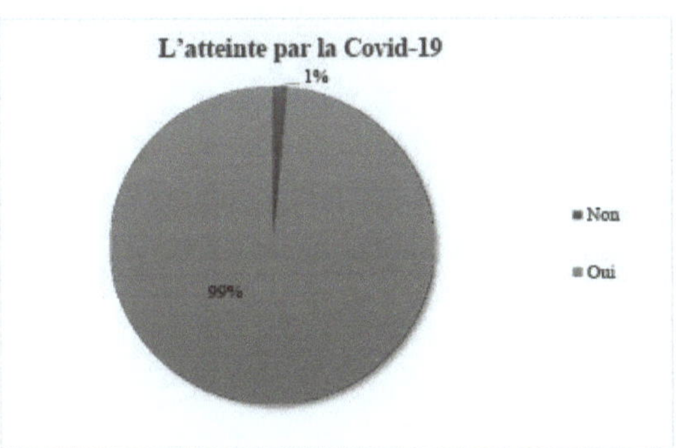

Figure 41: Distribution of the population according to Covid-19 status.

Half of the people who contracted Covid did so only once (166 people, i.e. 50%), while the others were reinfected with the virus two or more times (Table 13 and Figure 42).

Table 13: Distribution of people infected with Covid-19 according to the number of infections.

Number of Covid-19 infections	Workforce	Percentage
Only once	166	50%
Twice	114	35%
More than twice	50	15%
Total	330	100,00%

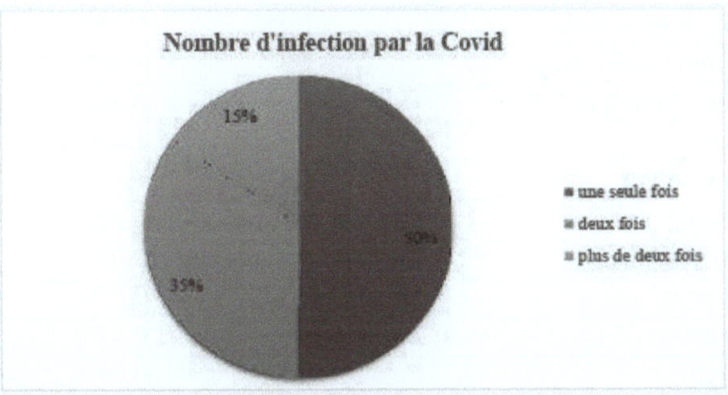

Figure 42: Rëpartition of people infected according to the number of infections.

• Breakdown of the population by Covid-19 symptoms

Fatigue, fever, headaches, aches and pains, coughing and loss of taste and smell were the most frequent symptoms in this study, in the following order: 13.8%, 13.5%, 12.9%, 11.86%, 9.69% and 9.36%. The remaining symptoms were diarrhoea (4.68%), breathing difficulties (4.4%) and nasal discharge (6.85%), while 28 people had suffered from asphyxia (1.32%). (Table 14, Figure 43).

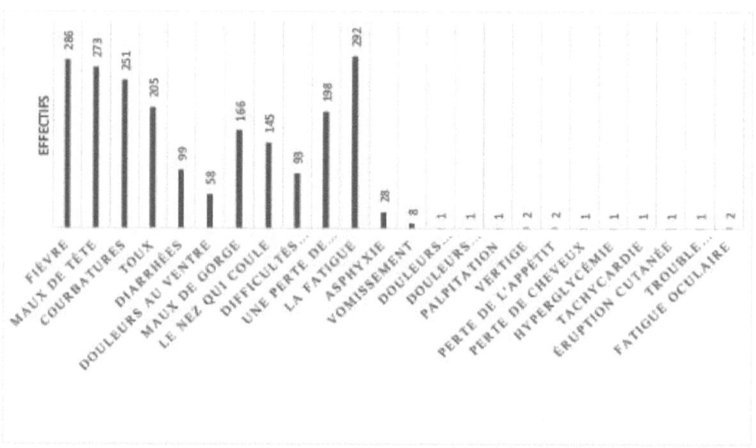

Figure 43: Distribution of people with coronavirus according to their symptoms.

Symptoms of Covid-19	Workforce	Percentage
Fever	286	13,52%
Headaches	273	12,90%
Curvature	251	11,86%
Cough	205	9,69%
Diarrhde	99	4,68%
Stomach pain	58	2,74%
Sore throats	166	7,84%
Runny nose	145	6,85%
Breathing difficulties	93	4,40%
A loss of smell or taste	198	9,36%
Fatigue	292	13,80%
Asphyxiation	28	1,32%
Vomiting	8	0,38%
Chest pain	1	0,05%
Joint pain	1	0,05%
Palpitation	1	0,05%
Vertigo	2	0,09%
Loss of appetite	2	0,09%
Hair loss	1	0,05%
Hyperglycaemia	1	0,05%
Tachycardia	1	0,05%
Skin rash	1	0,05%
Neurological disorders	1	0,05%
Eye fatigue	2	0,09%
Total	2116	100%

- Breakdown of people with Covid-19 by duration of symptoms

54

Among people with Covid-19, 29% had symptoms lasting from 1 to 5 days, 31% had symptoms lasting from 6 to 10 days, and 12% were unsure of the duration of their symptoms (Table 15, Figure 44).

Table 15: Rëpartition of people with Covid-19 by duration of symptoms.

Duration of Covid-19 symptoms	Workforce	Percentage
1-5 days	97	29%
6-10 days	103	31%
11-15 days	49	15%
16-20 days	22	7%
20 days to go	20	6%
I don't know	39	12%
Total	330	100%

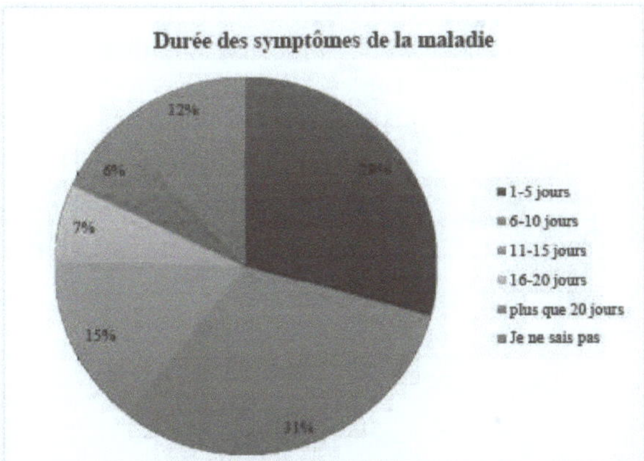

Figure 44: Duration of Covid-19 symptoms in the study population.

- Distribution of people according to the contagiousness of the virus

93% of those questioned said that there were other people around them who had been sickened by Covid-19 or had shown signs of the disease. (Table 16, figure 45)

Tableau 16: Rëpartition of people according to the presence of people ill with Sars-CoV- 2 in their entourage.

Other people infected with Covid	Number	Percentage
No	23	7%
Yes	312	93%
Total	335	100%

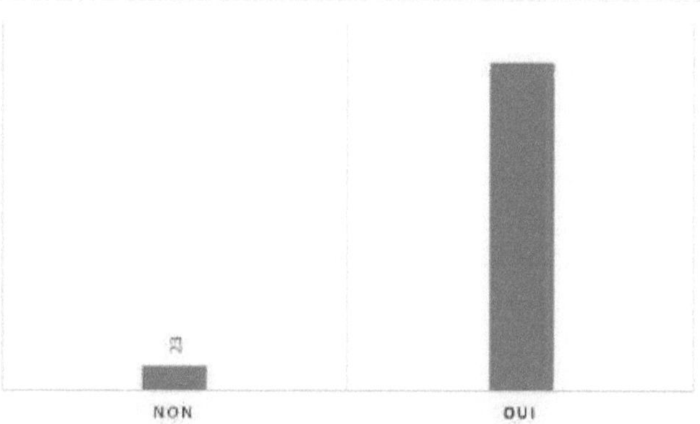

Figure 45: Rëpartition of people according to the presence of other people infected with Sars-CoV-2 in their entourage.

- Distribution of the population according to use of the coronavirus test

61% of those surveyed had used screening or diagnostic tests for the coronavirus, while 39% had not. (Table 17 and figure 46).

Tableau 17: Distribution of people by use of Covid tests.

Covid test	Number	Percentage
No	132	39%
Yes	203	61%
Total	335	100%

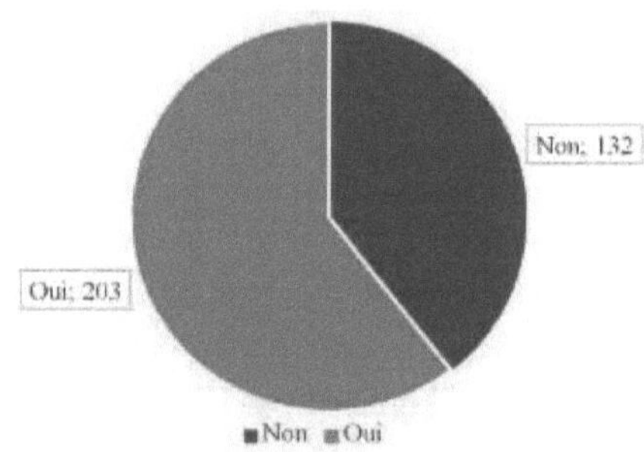

Figure 46: Distribution of people by use of Covid tests.

Of the people surveyed, 79 used antigenic tests (39%), while the remainder used RT-PCR and serological tests (18% and 21% respectively). Some people did all three types of test at the same time (Table 18 and Figure 47).

Table 18: Rëpartition of people according to the type of Covid test used.

Type of test	Workforce	Percentage
Antigen test	79	39%

PCR test	37	18%
PCR test, Antigen test	4	2%
PCR test, Serological test	9	4%
PCR test, Serological test, Antigen test	8	4%
Serological test	42	21%
Serological test, Antigen test	24	12%
Total	203	100%

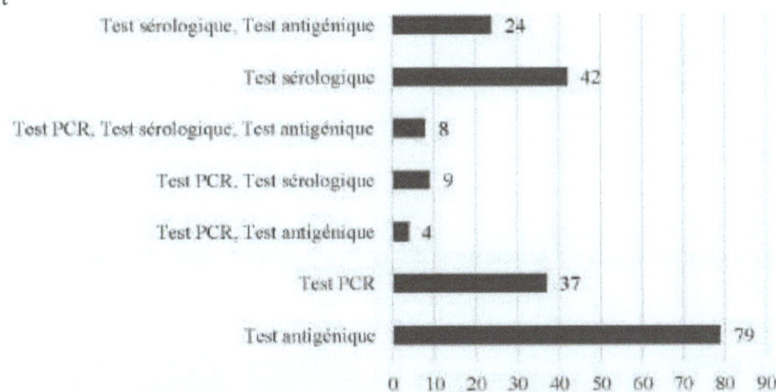

Figure 47: Répartition des personnes selon le type de test Covid utilisé.

- Breakdown of people by type of care
The percentage of people surveyed who had Covid-19 and who had requiring hospitalisation was only 5%. (Table 19, Figure 16)

Table 19: Breakdown of people by type of care.

Support	Number	Percentage
No	109	33%
Yes, I consulted a doctor	208	62%
Yes, I was hospitalised	18	5%
Total	335	100%

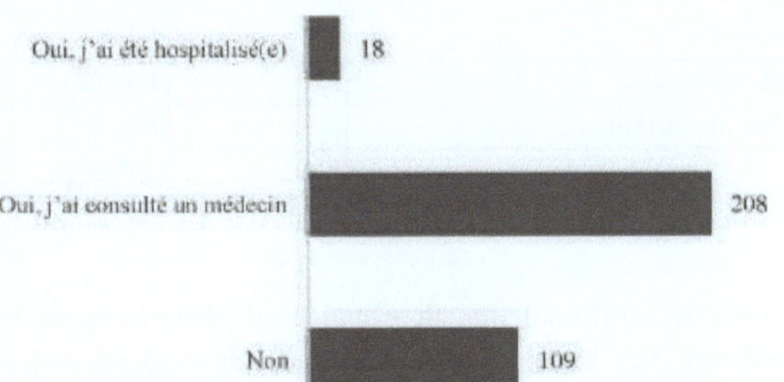

Figure 48: Rëpartition of people according to care.

- Breakdown of people by type of drug treatment

Vitamins (vitamin C, vitamin D, etc.) and mineral supplements (zinc, etc.) accounted for 23.05% of the treatments taken by respondents who had Covid-19, antibiotics (20.28%), chloroquine and hydroxychloroquine (1.01%) and 1.93% used no medication at all. (Table 20 and Figure 49).

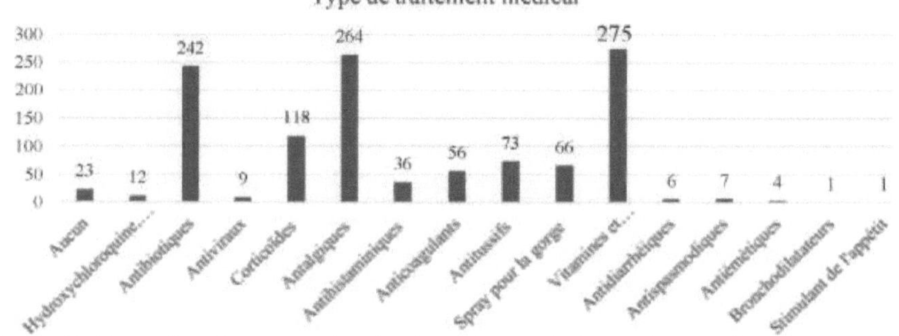

Figure 49: Type of mëdicaments taken by the study population against Covid-19.

Table 20: Frequency and percentage of medications taken for Covid-19

Treatment	Workforce	Percentage
No	23	1,93%
Hydroxychloroquine, Chloroquine	12	1,01%
Antibiotics	242	20,28%
Antivirals	9	0,75%
Corticoides	118	9,89%
Analgesics	264	22,13%
Antihistamines	36	3,02%
Anticoagulants	56	4,69%
Cough suppressants	73	6,12%
Throat spray	66	5,53%
Vitamins and mineral supplements	275	23,05%
AntidiaiTlieiques	6	0,50%
Antispasmodics	7	0,59%
Antiemetics	4	0,34%
Bronchodilators	1	0,08%
Appetite stimulant	1	0,08%
Total	1193	100,00%

- Distribution of the population according to the use of medicinal plants during treatment

83% of those questioned confirmed that they had used phytotherapies to prevent or cure Covid-19, while 17% of the population studied had not used phytotherapies during the pandemic. The table and diagram below report the number and frequency of people using phytotherapies to prevent or cure Covid-19. (Table 21 and figure 50)

Table 21: number and frequency of people with ийНзё phytotherapy against Covid- 19.

Use of phytotherapy	Workforce	Percentage
No	57	17%
Yes	278	83%
Total	335	100%

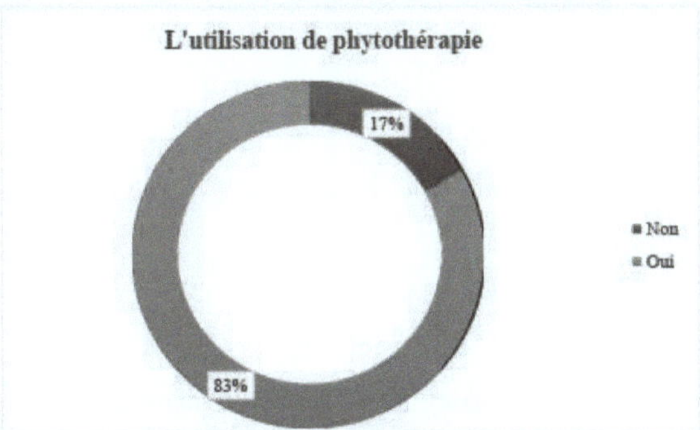

Figure 50: Distribution of people according to the use of phytotherapy.

Thyme, ginger, cloves and verbena were the plants most commonly used in the treatment of coronavirus disease, with percentages of 17.69%, 16.18%, 15.18% and 13.37%. (Table 21 and Figure 51).

Table 22: mёdicinal plants ийНзё during the Covid.

Medicinal plants	Workforce	Percentage
White mugwort	31	3,12%
Thyme	176	17,69%
Mint	127	12,76%
Vervain	133	13,37%
Eucalyptus	113	11,36%
Noble laurel	12	1,21%
Nigella cultivation	20	2,01%
Rosemary	37	3,72%
Ginger	161	16,18%
Cloves	151	15,18%
The onion	15	1,51%
Lemon	10	1,01%
Chamomile	3	0,30%
Cinnamon	1	0,10%
Aniseed	1	0,10%
Lavender	2	0,20%
The pistachio tree	1	0,10%
The Indian costus	1	0,10%
Total	995	100,00%

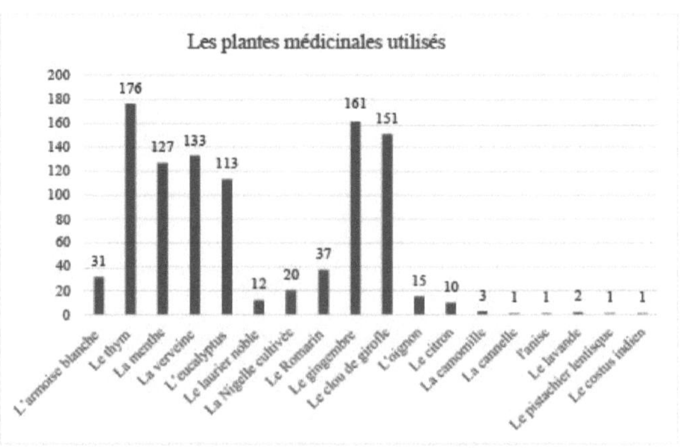

Figure 51: Frequency of mëdicinal plants ийНзё during Covid treatment.

- Rëpartition of the population according to receipt of Covid vaccine
More than half of the people surveyed had not received a vaccine against Covid-19 (210 people or 63%). (Table 23 and figure 52).

Table 23: Frequency of people who had or had not received a vaccine against covid-19.

Covid-19 vaccine	Workforce	Percentage
No	210	63%
Yes	125	37%
Total	335	100%

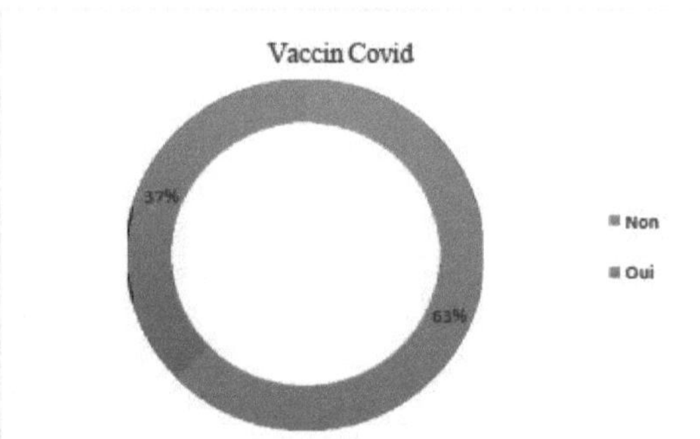

Figure 52: Distribution of the population according to receipt of Covid vaccine.

Of those vaccinated, 75% had received a vaccine called Coronavac from the sinovac laboratory. Followed by the vaxzevria vaccine (Astrazeneca) with a percentage of 12% and Sputnik V (6%). (Table 24 and Figure 53).
Table 24: Type of vaccine used against Covid-19.

Type of vaccine	Workforce	Percentage
I don't know	7	6%
Coronavac (Sinovac)	94	75%
Spikevax (Moderna)	1	1%
Sputnik V (Gamelya)	8	6%
Vaxzevria (Astrazeneca)	15	12%
Total	125	100%

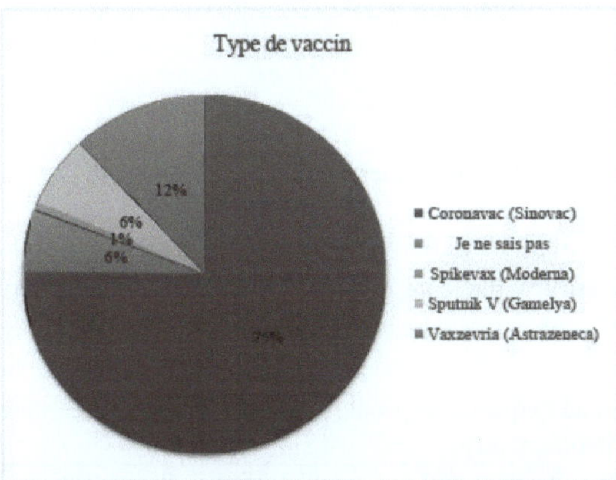

Figure 53: Distribution of vaccines according to the type of Covid vaccine used.

C. The organic and psychosocial sequelae of Sars-CoV-2

❖ Organic waste

• Distribution of people infected with Covid-19 according to the evolution of symptoms after the first week of infection

After the first week of infection with Sars-CoV-2, 82% of those infected said their symptoms had improved (270 people), while 18% (60 people) said their symptoms had worsened (Table 25 and Figure 54).

Table 25: Progression of symptoms after the first week of infection with Sars-CoV-2.

Development of symptoms after the first week of the disease	Workforce	Percentage
Addresses	270	81%
Aggravations	60	18%
Total	330	100%

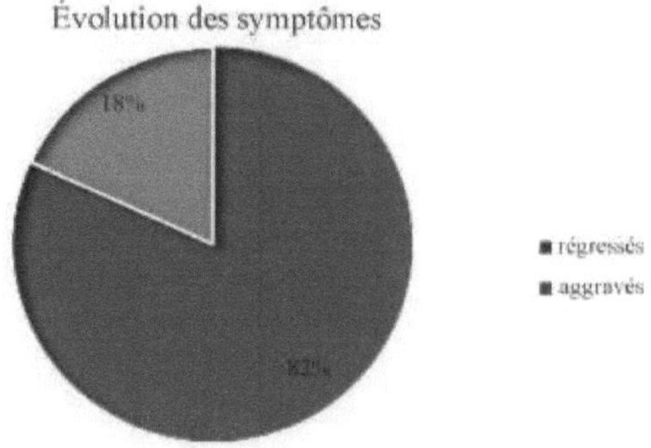

Figure 54: The evolution of symptoms after the first week of infection.

• **Breakdown of Covid-19 patients by recovery time**

The data from our survey indicate that 23% (76 people) need between 11 and 15 days, while only 9% of cases take more than 30 days to heal completely. (Table 26 and Figure 55)

Table 26: Percentage and frequency of people infected with Covid according to the length of time they have been in the country.

healing.

Time to heal	Workforce	Percentage
1-5 days	46	14%
6-10 days	65	20%
11-15 days	76	23%
16-20 days	47	14%
21-25 days	40	12%
26-30 days	26	8%
More than 30 days	30	9%
Total	330	100%

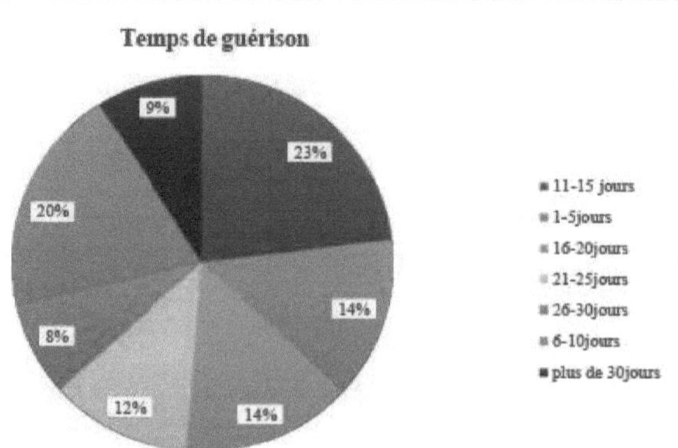

Figure 55: Distribution of people infected with Covid-19 according to recovery time.

62

- Distribution of the infected population according to persistence of symptoms
52% of people infected with Sars-CoV-2 (171 people) still have symptoms or
signs of the disease, while 48% gave a negative response. (Table 27 and Figure
56).

Tableau 27:   Percentage and frequency of persistence of Sars-CoV-2 symptoms.

Symptom of Covid long	Workforce	Percentage
Yes	171	52%
No	159	48%
Total	330	100%

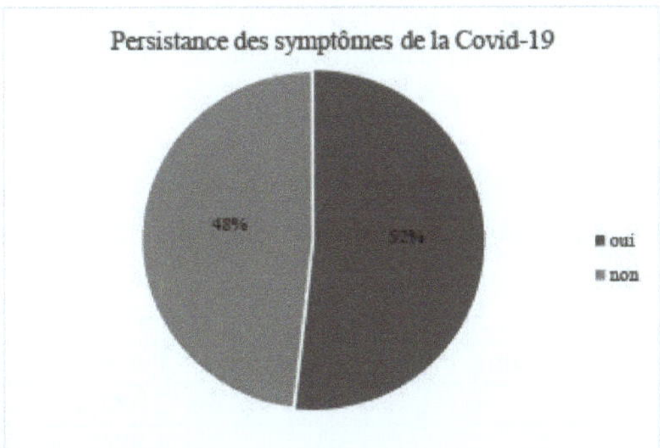

Figure 56: Distribution of people infected with Covid-19 according to persistence of
symptoms.

Breakdown of people by type of Covid long symptom

J General symptoms

Among the general symptoms of Covid long, fatigue is the most common,
accounting for 70% (100 people). (Table 28 and Figure 57).

Tableau 28:   Frequency and percentage of people with general symptoms of Covid long.

General symptoms	Workforce	Percentage
Fatigue	100	70%
Obesite	9	6%
Weight loss	35	24%
Total	144	100%

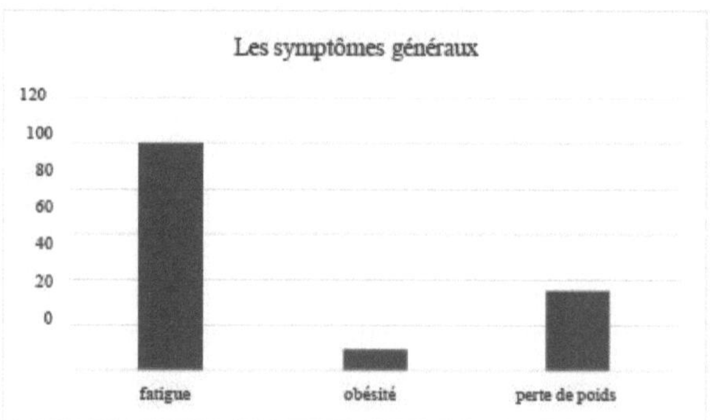

Figure 57: Distribution of people with general symptoms of Covid long.

Neurological symptoms

Among the neurological symptoms of long covid, memory and sleep disorders and dizziness were the most frequently cited by people with long covid symptoms (Table 29 and Figure 58).

Tableau 29:   Frequency and percentage of neurological symptoms in Covid long.

Neurological symptoms	Workforce	Percentage
Cdphaldes	35	21,88%
Epilepsy	3	1,88%
Sleep disorders	38	23,75%
Dizziness	38	23,75%
Memory disorders	44	27,50%
Migraine	2	1,25%
Total	160	100,00%

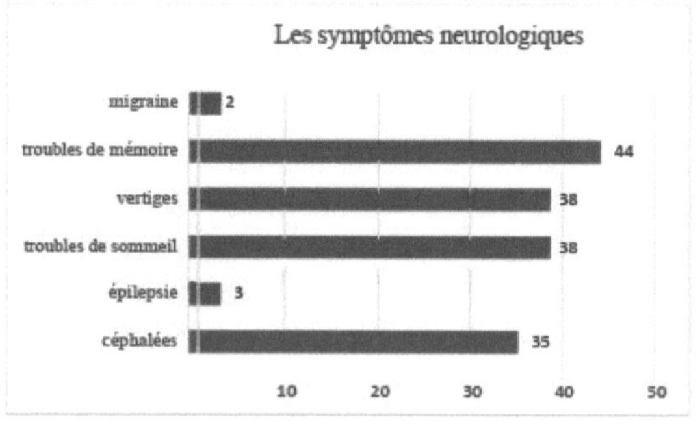

Figure 58: Distribution of people according to neurological symptoms of long covid.

Pulmonary symptoms

Among the pulmonary symptoms of Covid long, dyspnea was the most marked symptom among those questioned, with a percentage of 52.31%. (Table 30 and Figure 59).

Table 30: Frequency and percentage of pulmonary symptoms.

Respiratory symptoms	Workforce	Percentage
Dvspnee	34	52,31%
Asthma	10	15,38%
COPD	4	6,15%
Bronchial hyperventilation	8	12,31%
Persistent cough	7	10,77%
Chest tightness	1	1,54%
Recurrent upper respiratory tract infection	1	1,54%
Total	65	100,00%

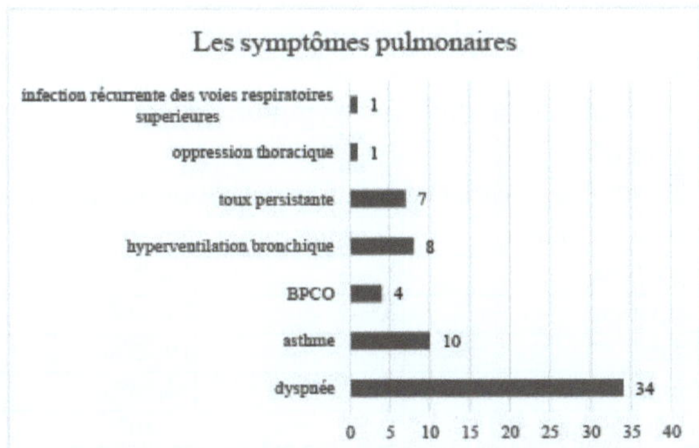

Figure 59: Frequency of pulmonary symptoms.

Cardiovascular symptoms

High blood pressure and arrhythmia are the most frequent cardiac symptoms with

percentages: 43.75% and 37.50. (Table 31 and Figure 60)

Table 31: Frequency and percentage of cardiovascular symptoms.

Cardiovascular symptoms	Workforce	Percentage
Arrhythmia	12	37,50%
HTA	14	43,75%
Heart failure	5	15,63%
Pdricarditis	1	3,13%
Total	32	100,00%

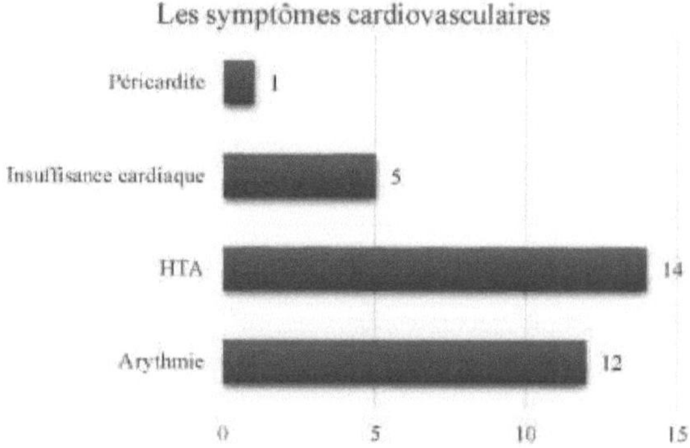

Figure 60: Frequency and percentage of cardiovascular symptoms.

Digestive symptoms

Gastritis was the most abundant digestive symptom, accounting for 28.40%. (Table 32 and Figure 61).

Table 32: Frequency and percentage of digestive symptoms.

Digestive symptoms	Workforce	Percentage
Irritable bowel	2	2,47%
Constipation	20	24,69%
Diarrhde	16	19,75%
Abdominal pain	20	24,69%
Gastritis (resophagitis...)	23	28,40%
Total	81	100,00%

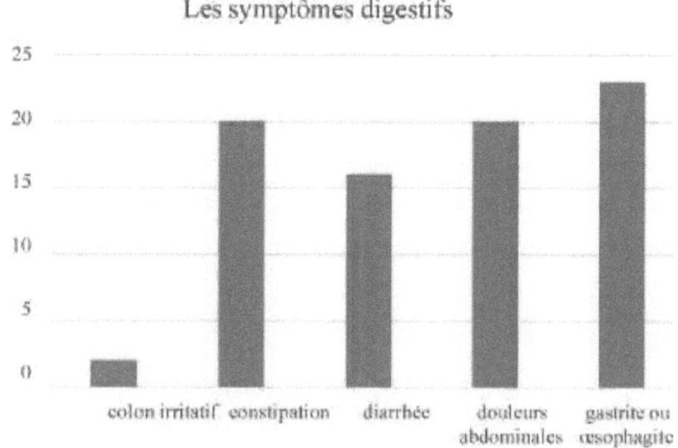

Figure 61: Frequency and percentage of digestive symptoms.

Musculo-tendinous and joint symptoms

Joint pain was the most frequent symptom with a percentage of 71.64% (Table 33 and Figure 62).

Table 33: Frequency and percentage of people with musculotendinous and articular symptoms.

Musculo-tendinous and joint symptoms	Workforce	Percentage
Joint pain	48	71,64%
Myalgia	19	28,36%
Total	67	100,00%

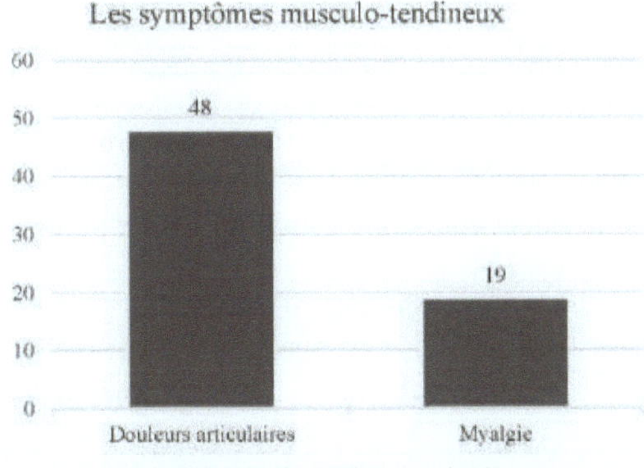

Figure 62: Frequency and percentage of musculotendinous and articular symptoms.

Eye symptoms

Decreased visual acuity and visual fatigue are the most frequent ocular symptoms of Covid long with the following percentages 43.75% and 42.19%. (Table 34 and Figure 63).

Table 34: Frequency and percentage of ocular symptoms.

Eye symptoms	Workforce	Percentage
Reduced visual acuity	28	43,75%
Eye pain	9	14,06%
Visual fatigue	27	42,19%
Total	64	100,00%

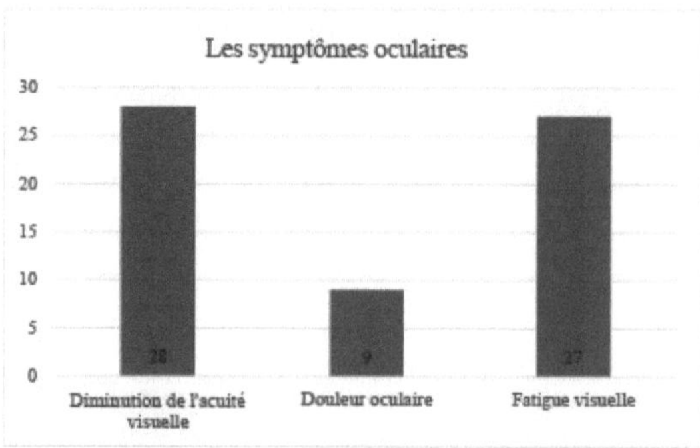

Figure 63: Frequency and percentage of ocular symptoms.

Endocrine symptoms

Diabetes is the most frequent endocrine symptom with a percentage of 66.67%. (Table 35 and figure 64)

Table 35: Frequency and percentage of endocrine symptoms.

Endocrine symptoms	Workforce	Percentage
Diabetes	12	66,67%
Thyroi'dite	6	33,33%
Total	18	100,00%

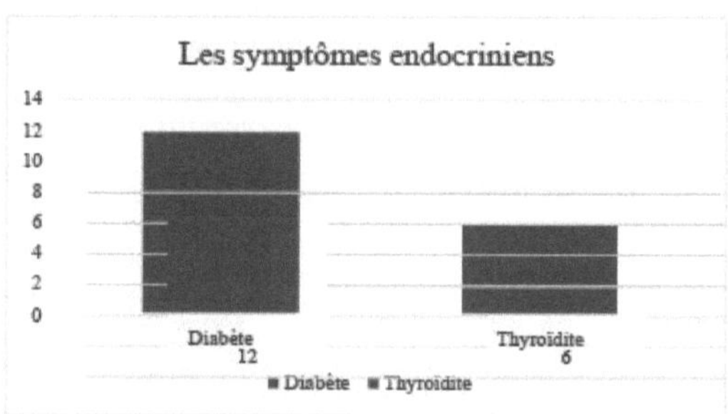

Figure 64: Frequency and percentage of endocrine symptoms.

Other symptoms

Among the other symptoms of long Covid, loss of taste and smell is the most frequently observed with a percentage of 48%. (Table 36 and figure 65)

Table 36: Frequency and percentage of other Covid long symptoms.

Other symptoms	Workforce	Percentage
Eczema	2	8%
Skin irritation	2	8%
Loss of appetite	1	4%
Loss of taste and smell	12	48%
Hair loss	1	4%
Skin dryness	1	4%
Coagulopathy	4	16%

Hypoglycemia	1	4%
Allergy	1	4%
Total	25	100%

Other symptoms of Covid long

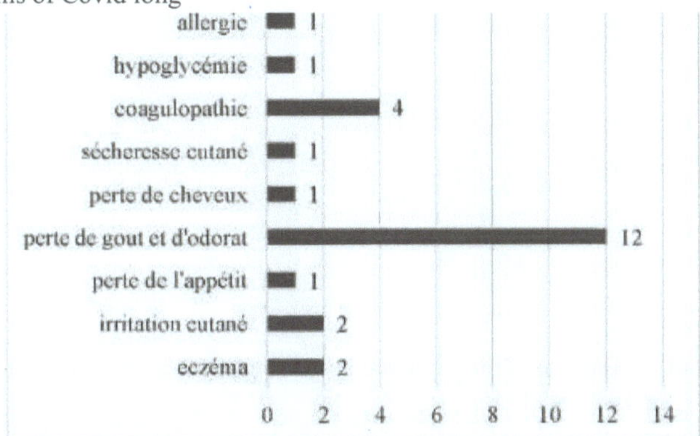

Figure 65: Fréquence et pourcentage d'autres symptômes de Covid long

❖ Psychic sequels

- Breakdown of the population by mental disorder prior to Covid-19

Of the people surveyed, 94% (314 people), the majority, did not have psychological problems before the Covid-19 pandemic, while 6% (21 people) did. (Table 37 and figure 66)

- Breakdown of the population by mental disorder during Covid

Among the respondents to our study, 75%, the majority of the population (251 people), did not have any psychiatric disorders during the Covid-19par pandemic, compared with 25% of the population who did (Table 38 and Figure 67). Anxiety and depression were the most frequent psychological disorders, with percentages in the following order: 24.86% and 20%. (Table 39 and Figure 68).

Tableau 37   : Rëpartition of the population according to the presence of psychological disorders during the Covid.

Presence of psychiatric disorders	Number	Percentage
No	251	75%
Yes	84	25%
Total	335	100,00%

Tableau 38   Breakdown of the population by mental disorder prior to Covid-19.

Psychological disorders before Covid 19	Workforce	Percentage
No	314	94%
Yes	21	6%

69

Total	335	100%

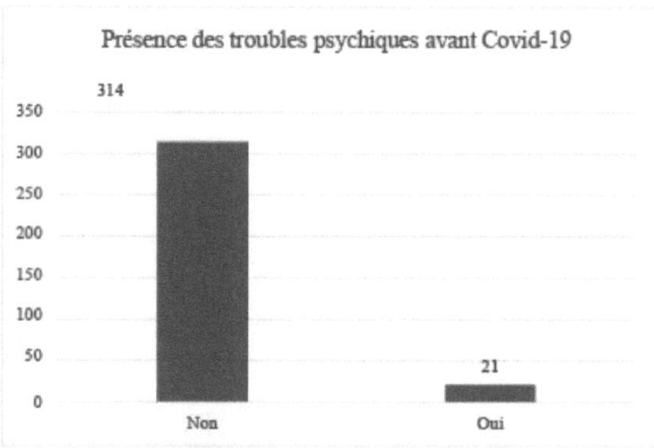

Figure 66: Breakdown of the population by mental disorder before Covid-19.

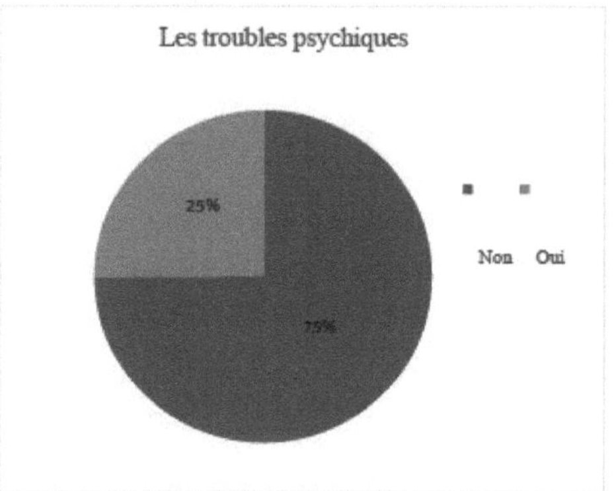

Figure 67: Rëpartition of population according to psychological disorders during Covid.
Table 39: Mental disorders during Covid-19.

Mental disorders	Workforce	Percentage
Anxiëtë	46	24,86%
Irritability	10	5,41%
Lack of concentration	33	17,84%
Depression	37	20,00%
Nervosite	22	11,89%
Panic disorder	13	7,03%
Phobia	13	7,03%
Schizophrenia	3	1,62%
TOC	4	2,16%
Insomnia	4	2,16%
Total	185	100,00%

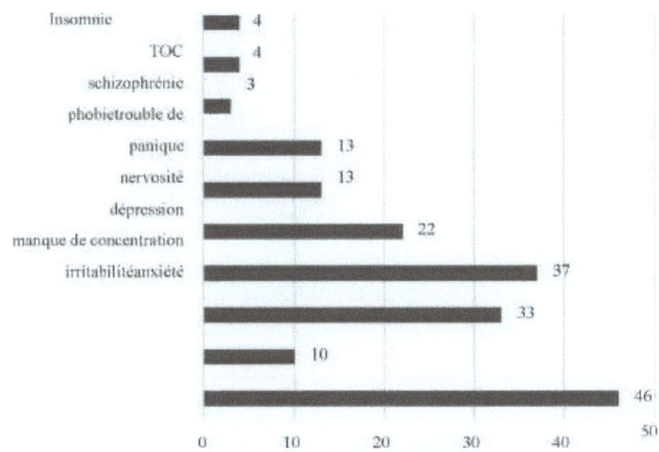

Figure 68: Mental disorders during Covid-19.

- Breakdown of the population by consumption of psychotropic drugs during the Covid

Of the people surveyed, 92% did not take any psychotropic drugs during the Covid, but only 8% did (Table 40, Figure 69).

Tableau 40   Distribution of the population according to consumption of psychotropic drugs during the Covid.

Consumption of psychotropic drugs	Workforce	Percentage
No	307	92%
Yes	28	8%
Total	335	100,00%

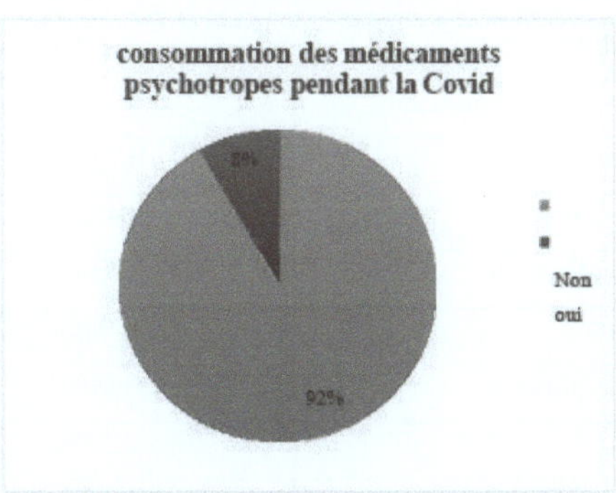

Figure 69: Breakdown of the population by use of psychotropic drugs during the Covid.

- Breakdown of the population according to psychological symptoms after Covid-19

Among the respondents to our study, the majority of the population (82%) had no psychological symptoms following the Covid-19 period, while 18% of the population (61 people) had psychological symptoms (Table 41 and Figure 70),

of which anxiety was the most frequent symptom with a percentage of 27.91%.
(Table 42 and Figure 71)

Tableau 41   Distribution of the population according to the presence of psychological
symptoms after the Covid-19 period.

The presence of psychological symptoms	Workforce	Percentage
No	274	82%
Yes	61	18%
Total	335	100%

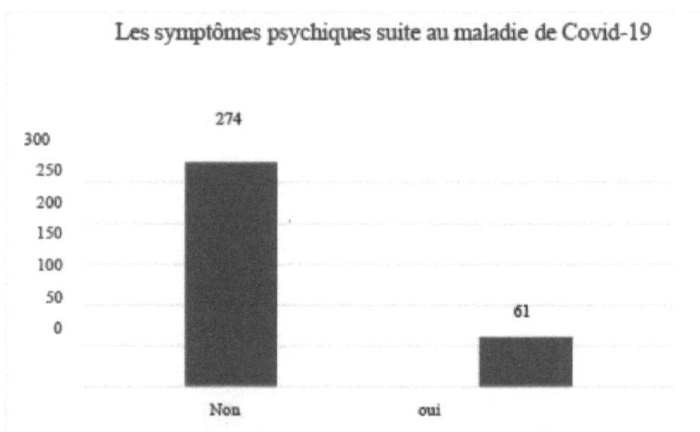

Figure 70: Distribution of the population according to the presence of psychological
symptoms following the Covid 19 period of depression.

Tableau 42   Types of psychological symptoms after Covid-19 illness

Mental disorders	Workforce	Percentage
Anxiëtë	36	27,91%
Irritability	7	5,43%
Lack of concentration	18	13,95%
Dëpression	22	17,05%
Nervosite	19	14,73%
Panic disorder	13	10,08%
Phobia	9	6,98%
Schizophrenia	0	0,00%
TOC	3	2,33%
Insomnia	2	1,55%
Total	129	100,00%

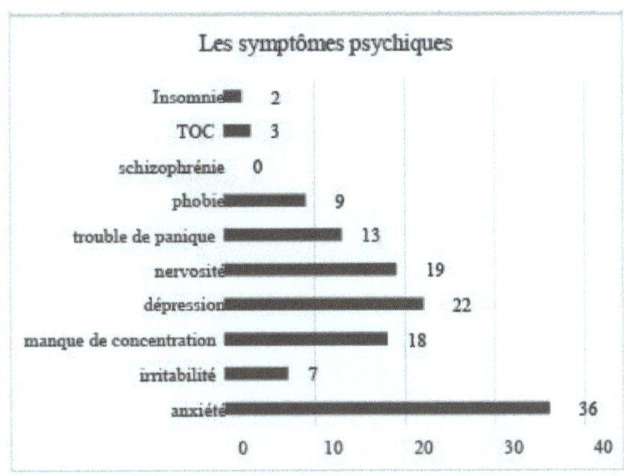

Figure 71: types of psychological symptoms after the Covid-19 përiod.

◆ Social after-effects

- Breakdown of the population according to cessation of daily life following Covid-19

66% of the population surveyed stopped their daily activities because of Covid-19. (Table 43 and figure 72).

Table 43: Percentage and frequency of people who had stopped or not stopped their daily activities following Covid-19.

The end of daily activities	Workforce	Percentage
No	113	34%
Yes	222	66%
Total	335	100,00%

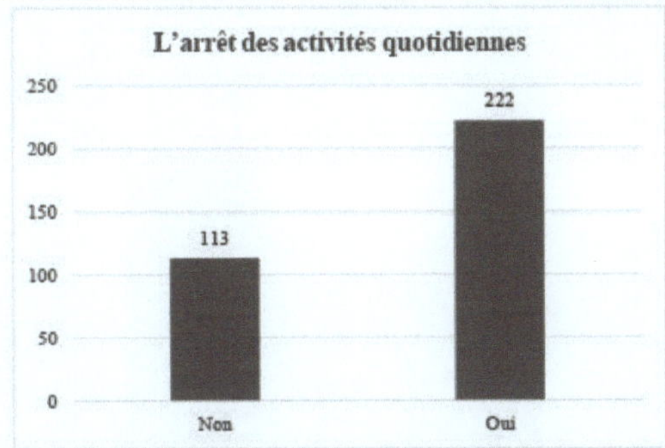

Figure 72: The impact of Covid 19 on people stopping their daily activities.

- Breakdown of the population by length of absence from work during Covid-19 The minority, i.e. 16% (26 people) of workers, stopped work definitively because of Covid-19 (Table 44 and Figure 73). Of these, 42% found other work (Table 45 and Figure 74), mainly in the state and private sectors, with a percentage of 45% for each. (Table 46 and Figure 75).

Table 44: Rëpartition of people according to whether they stopped working during the

pandëmia of the
Covid-19.

Work stoppage	Workforce	Percentage
Temporarily	76	46%
Definitely	26	16%
No	63	38%
Total	165	100,00%

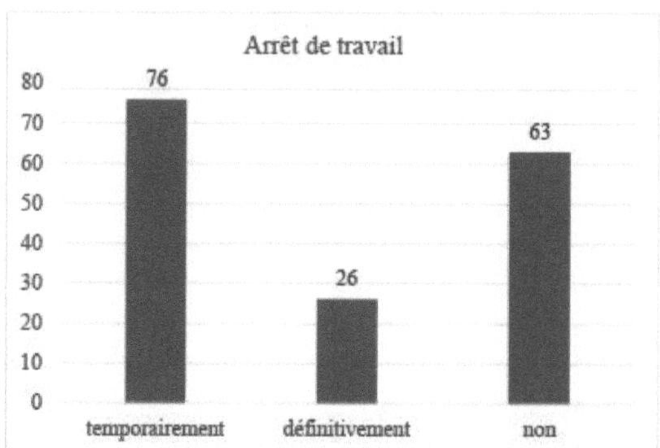

Figure 73: Distribution of the population according to time off work during the pandemic.

Table 45: Number and percentage of people finding other work.

New job	Workforce	Percentage
Yes	11	42%
No	15	58%
Total	26	100,00%

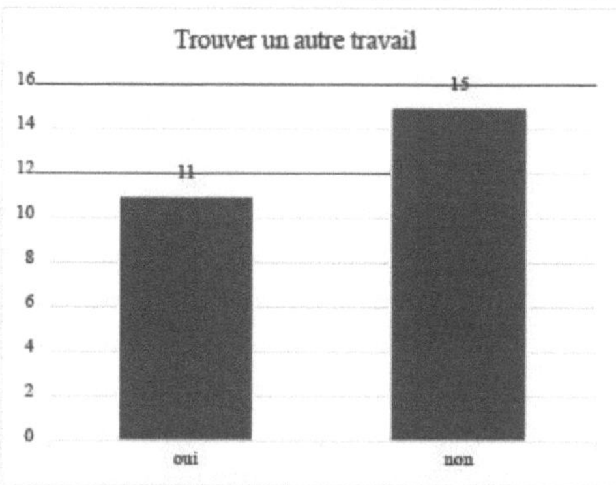

Figure 74: Number of people who found other work.

Table 46: Workforce and percentage of work areas

Area of work	Workforce	Percentage
Tëlëtravail	1	10%

State	5	45%
Private	5	45%
Total	11	100 %

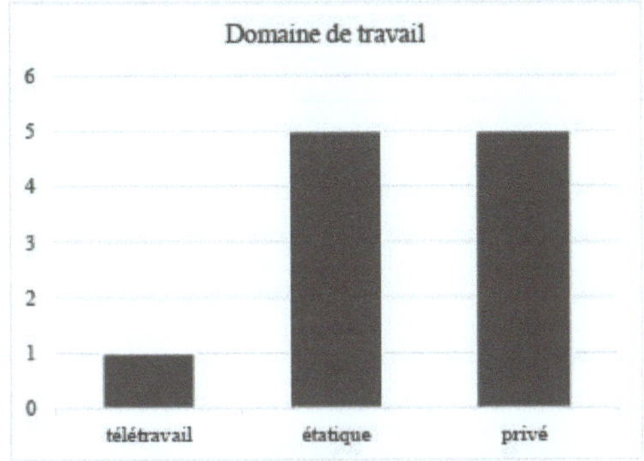

Figure 75: Workforce by area of work

- Breakdown of the population according to the end of education

Among the respondents to our study, the majority of the population (73% or 165 people) stopped their education during the Covid-19 pandemic, while 27% of the population did not (Table 47 and Figure 76).

Table 47: Distribution of the population according to the end of rehabilitation.

Education break	Workforce	Percentage
Yes	165	73%
No	62	27%
Total	227	100,00%

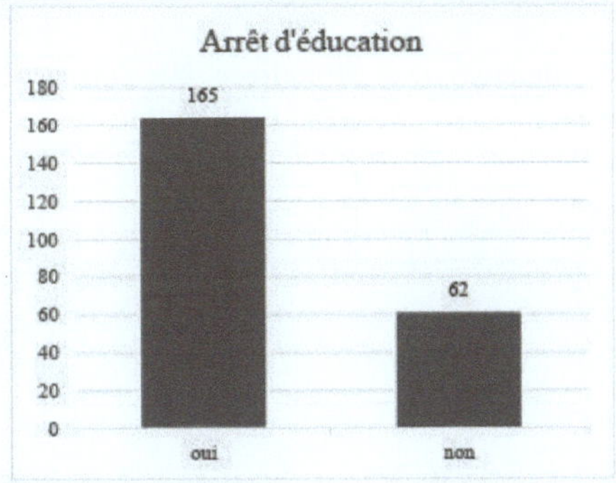

Figure 76 : Breakdown of the population according to cessation of rehabilitation.

- Breakdown of the population by financial situation :

More than half of the population surveyed 54% (182 people) were Qa will be financed during the Covid-19 period. (Table 48 and Figure 77)

Table 48: Breakdown of the population by financial situation.

Financially :	Number	Percentage
Qa va	182	54%
You were at ease	66	20%
You can't do it without going into debt.	12	4%
It's hard to do	75	22%
Total	335	100%

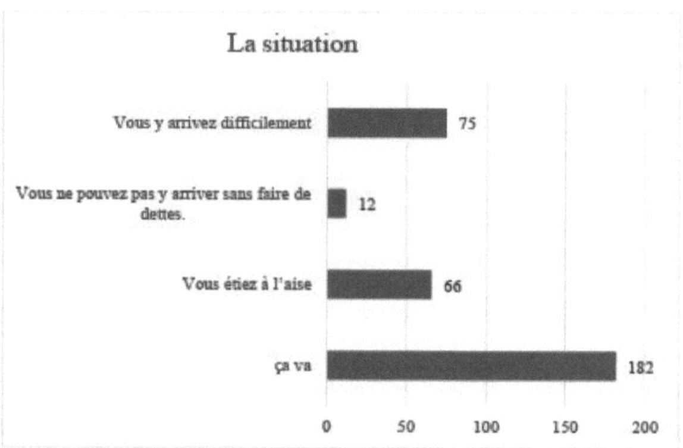

Figure 77: Rëpartition of the population by financial situation.

- Distribution of the population according to the impact of Covid-19 on family situation :

Covid-19 had no impact on family situation for the majority of the population (97%). (Table 49 and figure 78)

Table 49: Distribution of the population according to the impact of Covid 19 on family situation

Family situation	Workforce	Percentage
No impact	324	97%
Manage	8	2%
Divorce	3	1%
Total	335	100%

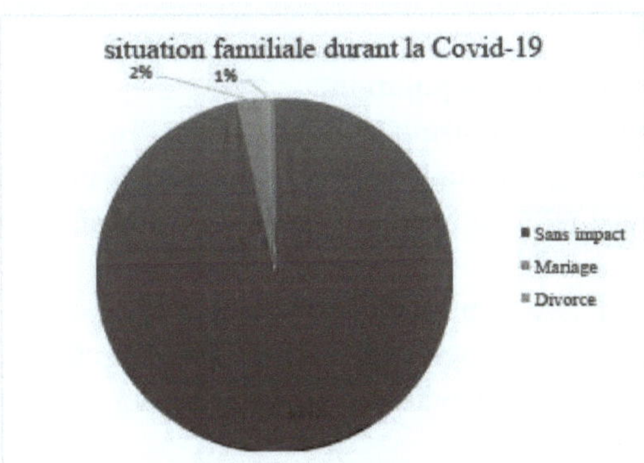

Figure 78: Rëpartition of the population according to 1 impact of Covid-19 on family situation.

- Breakdown of the population by number of new births during the Covid :

Among 116 people married before the Covid period, 43% (50 people) had children during the Covid-19 pandemic, and 57% gave a negative response. (Table 50 and figure 79).

Table 50: Breakdown of population by number of new births

New birth	Workforce	Percentage
Yes	50	43%
No	66	57%
Total	116	100 %

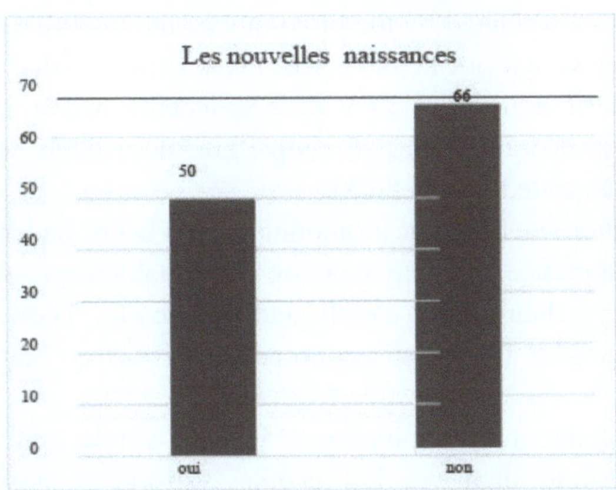

Figure 79: Rëpartition of the population according to the number of new births.

VI.3.3. Discussion

A. Descriptive data on the population

Our study was carried out using a questionnaire intended for the general population, representing 335 individuals. There was a clear predominance of women (72%) compared with men (28%), giving a female-to-male sex ratio of 2.56.

According to a study by San Jose State University, it has been shown that women are more likely to participate in online surveys than men [128]. As with traditional survey methods, women respond in higher proportions than men. [129]

Women may be more comfortable with communication and feel more confident in expressing their opinions; in addition, they may be more motivated to share their ideas and experiences, particularly on subjects that concern them directly.

The age range of study was from under 18 to over 50. The majority (62%) were in the 18-30 age group.

Young people are more active in the surveys than older people. There may be several reasons for this: young people may have more free time and greater flexibility in their schedules, which makes it easier for them to take part in surveys. Young people, on the other hand, may have family commitments, work responsibilities or health problems that limit their availability to take part in surveys. Older people may be less comfortable with technology and less likely to use the Internet.

Of the 335 respondents, the inhabitants of El Taref and Annaba were the most likely to reply to the questionnaire, with percentages of 34% and 32% respectively. This is explained by the proximity of the interviewers and the fact that these are large wilayas located in border areas with Tunisia.

As for the level of education, 77% of respondents had a higher level of education. In general, more educated people are more likely to participate in surveys than less educated people [128].

People with a higher level of education often have a better understanding of the survey and its importance, and may be more comfortable expressing themselves and communicating their views clearly and coherently. They may be better equipped to understand the questions posed in the survey and provide more detailed answers.

More than half of the study population (65%) are single. Single people may have more free time than married people, especially those with family responsibilities.

In terms of socio-professional category, 50% of survey respondents were students, reflecting the highest age bracket in our survey.

78% of our respondents did not have a chronic illness, which explains why the majority of young subjects were in good health and had no underlying illnesses (91%).

According to the WHO, heart disease remains the main cause of death; diabetes and dementia are in the top 10 [130]. In our survey, cardiovascular disease and diabetes predominated, accounting for 26% and 22% respectively of all chronic diseases.

B. Involvement and treatment of Covid-19

99% of the people questioned had been affected by Covid-19 (Figure 41 and Figure 45). The Sars-CoV-2 responsible for the contagious disease Covid-19, The number of confirmed cases in Algeria, up to 19 May 2023, is 271,751 and 6881 deaths. [131]

There is an increased risk of reinfection by Covid-19, especially with the omicron variant [132]. According to the study by Xiangying Ren, Jie zhou and others, the sequence of viral genes revealed that some patients were reinfected by different strains and others by the same strains [133]. This was confirmed in our study, in which 50% of those questioned were infected twice or more with Covid-19.

Analysis of the symptomatological picture provided by our surveys revealed that the majority of patients experienced the following evocative symptoms, in order of incidence: asthenia or unusual fatigue (13.8%), fever (13.52%), and cough (9.69%).

According to Douard and Jean-Francois, most cases of Covid-19 present as pneumopathies, with aspecific symptoms: cough, fever, dyspnoea, rhinorrhea, pharyngitis and chest pain. Cephalalgia, myalgias, chills and sweats have also been reported. [134]

Among people with Covid-19, 31% had symptoms lasting between 6 and 10 days. Most of these people had mild to moderate symptoms, which generally disappeared after 1 to 2 weeks.

In our survey, 39% detected the disease using antigenic tests for several reasons: rapid results, ease of use and they are often less expensive than PCR tests.

62% of those surveyed consulted a doctor for diagnosis and confirmation of the disease through clinical examinations and screening tests, to assess the severity of symptoms, to obtain advice on managing these symptoms at home and to obtain advice on self-isolation and prevention measures to avoid transmitting the virus to others.

Most people take vitamins and mineral supplements, painkillers and antibiotics. Certain vitamin supplements, such as vitamin C, vitamin D, zinc and antioxidants, are known for their role in strengthening the immune system, their antioxidant properties and for acting on certain symptoms of Covid-19, such as fatigue and muscle soreness. Analgesics are used for the symptomatic treatment of the disease, and the use of antibiotics has tended to decrease after a few weeks of practice, due to the rarity of bacterial superinfections of Covid-19. [134]

83% of those questioned confirmed that they had used medicinal plants during their Covid-19 treatment. And 9a explained that traditional medicine, and especially phytotherapy, is considered as a complementary treatment to conventional treatment.

Cloves, thyme and ginger together accounted for 49% of the medicinal plants used by respondents with Covid-19 to treat the disease. (Figure 51) A study carried out by Ali Nadi and his colleagues showed that thyme (*Thymus Vulgaris*) was effective against Covid-19, and could suppress TNF-alpha, IL-6 and other inflammatory cytokines.

Thyme extract also acts as an inhibitor of both IL-1-beta and IL- 8 cytokines. [135]

63% of people surveyed are not vaccinated against Covid-19 because of misinformation and false beliefs about Covid-19 vaccines. In addition, some people may have doubts about the safety and efficacy of these vaccines. Our results are confirmed by a Tunisian study in 2022. [136]

A total of 75% of people vaccinated against Covid had received a vaccine called Coronavac developed by Sinovac, and Vaxzevria (Astrazeneca) came second with 12%. Firstly, production of anti-Covid vaccines began in September 2021 in Algeria, with the first doses of "CoronaVac", the Algerian version of the Chinese vaccine Sinovac in order to speed up the national vaccination campaign. [137]

Secondly, the AstraZeneca/Oxford vaccine is the most widely distributed in the world, since it is administered in three quarters of the countries and territories that vaccinate [138]. This two-injection vaccine has the advantage of being able to be stored in a simple refrigerator. [139]

The Agence nationale de securite du medicament confirmed the existence of a "rare" risk of atypical thrombosis associated with this vaccine, while emphasising that its benefit/risk balance remained "favourable". [140]

C. Organic and psychosocial sequelae of Sars-CoV-2

- Organic waste

After the first week of infection with Sars-CoV-2, 82% of those infected said that their symptoms had improved. According to our study, most of the Covid-19 cases were acute and mild, did not present chronic illnesses and had benefited from medical treatment to alleviate their symptoms.

According to the WHO, most people who contract the Covid-19 virus recover without special treatment and in about two weeks. Although some suffer "long-term effects on several body systems, including the pulmonary, cardiovascular and nervous systems, as well as psychological effects" [141]. This is similar to our study, in which the complete recovery time was between 11 and 15 days for 23% of people, while only 9% of cases took more than 30 days.

According to Dominique Salmon and colleagues, approximately 25-30% of patients with an initial symptomatic form of Covid-19 still have symptoms 1 to 2 months after their initial diagnosis, and 10-15% at 6-8 months. Women were the most affected [142], which is consistent with our study. 52% of people infected with Covid-19 still have symptoms or signs of the disease, with women predominating (69%).

According to the HAS and Jessica SeeBle et al's cohort of German patients, one of the factors associated with prolonged forms of Covid-19 is female gender[143][144].

Fatigue was the most common symptom in our study, accounting for 70%. According to the WHO, fatigue is the most prevalent symptom [145], which may or may not be associated with other symptoms and a sensation of a sudden lack of energy (post-exertional malaise). [146]

According to Dominique Salmon Ceron, this is a form of fatigue that persists after the initial episode or reappears abruptly in waves after a phase of improvement. This fatigue, which is often major, can lead to exhaustion and a substantial reduction in everyday, professional, social and personal activities [142]. These studies confirm our findings.

According to Dominique, the main neurological symptoms encountered during Covid Long are cephalalgia, generally of the tensive type, often posterior, uni- or bilateral, cognitive disorders, sensory disorders, dizziness and sleep disorders. [142]

Similarly, the HAS reports that sleep disorders in long Covid may include insomnia, sleep fragmentation, the onset of nightmares and hypersomnia [147]. The distribution of post-acute Covid-19 disorders also includes neurocognitive manifestations such as concentration problems, attention problems (bradypsychia) and immediate memory problems, with a percentage of 45.1% according to the study by Dominique Salmon Ceron [146]. This confirms the results of our study.

Dyspnea is the most frequent pulmonary symptom of Covid long. This finding is consistent with that of other studies, such as the post-Covid-19 perspectives study by Damienet and colleagues (2022) in France at the Amiens-Picardie University Hospital: persistent symptoms after Covid-19 infection vary

[148][149]. In terms of respiratory symptoms, dyspnoea, particularly exertional dyspnoea, is the most common.
[150]
In our study we noted two peaks in cardiovascular symptoms
Post Covid-19: hypertension and arrhythmias this can be justified by the frequency of cardiovascular disease in Algeria even before the Covid period according to figure 40. According to D. SAUMON CERON and colleagues, cardio-thoracic symptoms include, in order of frequency, dyspnea, tachycardia and chest pain [151].

Tachycardia has been shown to be a common symptom associated with long Covid, with 25-50% of patients in a post-Covid tertiary multidisciplinary team clinic reporting persistent tachycardia or palpitations. [152]

According to an American study involving more than 150,000 infected patients, people who have contracted Covid-19 have a 55% increased risk of developing a cardiovascular disorder in the year following infection. More specifically, those affected were 72% more likely to have coronary heart disease, 63% more likely to have a heart attack and 52% more likely to have a stroke. [153]

Gastritis is the most abundant digestive symptom, which was a very frequent symptom even before Covid, due to the poor eating habits of the Algerian population and the stressful lifestyle, followed by digestive pain, constipation and diarrhoea, which was underestimated by the Algerian population because they did not make the link between diarrhoea and Covidlong. However, according to the HAS, chronic diarrhoea is the most frequent digestive symptom of long-Covid (around 6-10% of patients). [154]

Our survey showed that joint pain is the most frequent symptom of Covid long, followed by myalgia. This pain may be due to inflammation, tendonitis or arthritis.

According to HUG, muscle pain occurs twelve months after infection with Sars-CoV-2 in 7.3% of cases and joint pain in 3% of cases. [155]

A large published Canadian study found that muscle and joint pain were among the main symptoms reported [156]. The results of this study are consistent with several other studies around the world. [157]

According to Lolona Ramanantsoa, a general practitioner, the symptoms of long Covid include eye problems: tearing, eye fatigue and blurred vision [158]. In our survey, reduced visual acuity was the most frequent symptom, followed by eye fatigue.

The results of the survey revealed that diabetes is the most common endocrine symptom observed, enabling us to establish that Covid-19 is diabetogenic.

Studies have also shown that, as well as causing lung damage, Covid-19 appears to be responsible for the onset of diabetes in a number of healthy subjects: according to the work of Liu et al, 17% of their patients with severe Covid-19 had pancreatic lesions. They also reported that the pancreas is very rich in ACE2, a protein expressed in the two exocrine glands and the Hots of the pancreas and used as a viral entry point. The level of ACE2 expression is slightly higher in the pancreas. This suggests that Sars-CoV-2 may bind to ACE2 in the pancreas of non-diabetic individuals, destroying its cells and causing diabetes in these individuals. Sars-CoV-2 would therefore be diabetogenic. The authors believe that it may aggravate systemic inflammation, play a role in the development of respiratory distress syndrome ждиё and even cause chronic pancreatitis. [159]

A global analysis conducted in 2020 by Thirunavukkarasu Sathish, a population health researcher at McMaster University in Canada, showed that 15% of patients with a severe form of Covid-19 also developed diabetes. However, he admits that "this number is probably higher in people at risk, such as pre-diabetics". A study conducted in 2021 by Paolo Fiorina, an endocrinologist at Harvard Medical School, reported that of 551 patients hospitalised following Covid-19 in Italy, almost half became hyperglycemic. [160]

Loss of taste and smell is the most common symptom observed during and after Covid according to figure 65. According to a review by Nanki Hura BS of 552 initial candidate articles, 36 studies with data for 2183 patients with post-viral olfactory dysfunction. [161]

In another study of 292 patients who consulted for prolonged symptoms, anosmia/dysgeusia was the 10th most frequent Covidlong symptom. [162]

According to a British study published in the scientific journal *The Lancet*, only 17% of patients infected with Omicron lost their sense of taste and smell (compared with 53% with the Delta variant) [163]. This allows us to conclude that the Delta variant is the major cause of loss of taste and smell.

- Psychic effects

Compared to the pre-Covid period, the frequency of psychological disorders increased, as shown in Figures 66 and 67, with anxiety and depression being the most frequent symptoms (Figure 68).

A number of difficulties during this period were conducive to the onset of these symptoms, including: confinement, the loss of family members, psychological suffering linked to the illness of a close relative, especially an elderly one, and all the ensuing medical problems, poor patient care, shortages of heavy medication and oxygen, and the saturation of medical facilities, especially during unpredictable peaks. For others, the problem of temporary or permanent sick leave was the main cause of their suffering.

During the pandemic, when the world faced a halt or slowdown in daily activities and social distancing was practised to reduce inter-human interactions, healthcare professionals generally went in the opposite direction. With demands for healthcare growing exponentially, they are faced with long shifts, often with insufficient resources and unstable infrastructures.

In addition, many professionals may feel ill-prepared, especially as there is insufficient data on the virus and no well-established protocol or treatment for clinical interventions in patients infected with this new virus, as well as 9a concern about self-inoculation and the possibility of transmitting the virus to family, friends or colleagues. These factors can lead to various psychological disorders, such as stress, irritability and anxiety.

In 2020, previous studies have shown that epidemics and outbreaks of disease are followed by drastic psychosocial impacts, which end up becoming more pervasive than the epidemic itself. As a result of this pandemic, high levels of anxiety, stress and depression have already been observed in the general population. [163]

A meta-analysis of 19 studies (11,324 patients) reported, 3-6 months after the initial episode, an incidence of 23% for anxiety symptoms and 12% for depressive symptoms. [165]

Despite the significant incidence of mental health problems during the Covid, only 8% of those surveyed had taken psychotropic medication, for a number of reasons: Some people prefer to manage their mental health problems without medication and choose to focus on coping techniques and lifestyle changes to manage their symptoms. In addition, they prefer to avoid the heavy side-effects of psychotropic medication.

After the Covid-19 period, the frequency of mental disorders declined. This can be attributed to the almost total disappearance of the disease and the lifting of confinement by the government. As a result, people resumed their normal lives.

Despite the reduction in these disorders, they do not disappear completely and 9a remains Covid long mask and the most frequent symptom still remains l'anxiete.

- Social issues

Because of Covid-19, the majority of the population surveyed stopped their daily activities following the compulsory and necessary containment which was aimed at protecting public health and limiting the spread of the pandemic by putting in place numerous measures to avoid gatherings such as the closure of public establishments (nurseries, libraries, sports halls...), the restriction of international and national travel, the cancellation of events (concerts, festivals, conferences...).

Since March 2020, the coronavirus pandemic (Covid-19) has led to significant changes in the daily lives of individuals and communities. The application of health measures, such as closing schools and reducing social contacts, has led to upheavals in interpersonal relationships as well as in the spheres of work and study[166].

A large proportion of the population stopped work temporarily, especially during the lockdown. However, a minority stopped work permanently, with many industries affected by closures and social distancing measures, resulting in a large number of job losses in sectors such as hotels, restaurants, travel and tourism.

The self-employed and casual workers are also particularly affected, as are workers in the events and entertainment sector: cancellations of events and closures of theatres, cinemas and theme parks have had a devastating impact on workers in this sector, including artists, technicians and security guards.

While some patients return to a normal life within a few months, others continue to be off work because attempts to return to work too quickly are often unsuccessful. According to the follow-up cohort of patients who consulted us for prolonged symptoms, while only 5% had been hospitalised for the Covid-19 initial, one year later, only 50% had returned to work full-time, 30% had been able to return to work part-time, while 20% had not been able to return to work. [167]

Among those who lost their jobs permanently, some found other work, especially in the state or private sector (Figure 73), and teleworking was the least affected, unlike in other countries such as Canada (Figure 74). This situation reflects the Algerian population's lack of culture in this area compared with other countries.

According to Tremblay and his colleagues, new ways of working and collaborating between colleagues and between organisations have also been developed in several sectors in Canada. The use of telework and videoconferencing is the prime example, but other new practices may also emerge. [168,169]

Following the pandemic, education came to a standstill in several countries, including Algeria, and many countries closed their schools for extended periods. This led to major disruptions in student learning.

The lack of concentration associated with distance learning was also reported, with one student saying that he had to work much harder to pay attention. Students from programmes where practical work is an integral part of the training (e.g. firefighters, physiotherapists) were also affected because the online courses did not allow for the practical component. [166]

The majority of the population were financially well off, and the fact that they were able to rest during the Covid meant that some of them were able to manage their time and budget well.
It should be noted that there was an increase in births during the pandemic. This increase can be explained by the fact that some people spent more time at home due to remote working and confinement, which may have encouraged conception.

Conclusion

Covid-19 is an infectious disease caused by the new Sars-Cov-2 virus, which has spread rapidly around the world and is transmitted directly or indirectly between people.

The pandemic has had a considerable impact on the world's population since it emerged at the end of 2019. The pandemic has had major consequences for the physical, mental and social health of those affected.

The coronavirus can cause a range of symptoms, from mild to severe and even fatal. However, it is important to note that some individuals can be infected asymptomatically, which makes the spread of the virus all the more difficult to control.The results of the survey show that the vast majority of people questioned have been affected by the disease or have had close relatives affected. In addition, there is an increased risk of infection, particularly with the omicron variant. The most frequently observed symptoms are fatigue, fever, cough, sore throat, breathing difficulties and loss of taste or smell.

The duration of symptoms varies, but most people experience mild to moderate symptoms which generally disappear after 1 to 2 weeks.

Medical management often involves consultation with a doctor for diagnosis, clinical examinations and advice on symptom management and preventive measures. Common treatments include vitamins, mineral supplements, analgesics and antibiotics. In addition, many people resort to phytotherapy, using medicinal plants such as cloves, thyme and ginger.

The health impact of the Covid-19 pandemic has generally been tracked by reporting the number of cases, hospitalisations and deaths. But death is not the only major negative consequence of Sars-CoV-2 infection. It has become increasingly clear that many patients, even those with mild cases, can develop long-lasting symptoms that can have disabling consequences for those affected. These patients report a wide variety of symptoms.

The organic and psychosocial sequelae caused by the Sars-CoV-2 virus are persistent and complex problems, leading to a significant reduction in daily activities.

Organic sequelae include a variety of symptoms that can last for several months or even longer. Among the persistent symptoms, fatigue is the most frequently reported, followed closely by neurological symptoms such as cephalalgia, cognitive impairment and sleep disorders. As far as pulmonary symptoms are concerned, dyspnea, particularly during exertion, is a predominant symptom in people with long-standing Covid.

Cardiovascular symptoms such as hypertension and arrhythmias can be exacerbated after infection with Covid-19, and patients who contracted Covid-

19 had an increased risk of developing cardiovascular disorders such as coronary heart disease, heart attack and stroke.

Gastritis, digestive pain, constipation and diarrhoea are the most frequently observed digestive symptoms.

Musculo-tendinous symptoms are also present, particularly joint and muscle pain. These pains can be attributed to inflammation, tendonitis or arthritis.

The results of the survey reveal that diabetes is a frequent symptom in patients with long-standing covid, indicating that the disease has a diabetogenic effect, and that covid is the cause of the onset of diabetes in several healthy subjects.

Ocular symptoms have also been observed in some patients.

In addition, loss of taste and smell is a common symptom during and after Covid-19, particularly with the Delta variant.

The psycho-social after-effects are also a cause for concern, with an increase in the frequency of mental disorders such as anxiety and depression. Contributing factors include confinement, loss of loved ones, psychological suffering linked to a relative's illness, poor medical care and socio-economic difficulties such as loss of employment.

The Covid-19 pandemic has had an impact on every aspect of daily life. Mandatory containment measures have meant that people have had to stop their usual activities. In terms of employment, many jobs were temporarily or permanently lost, particularly in sectors such as hotels, restaurants and tourism. Some long-standing Covid patients have also found it difficult to return to full-time work because of prolonged symptoms.

Education has also been severely disrupted, with the closure of schools and the adoption of distance learning, leading to learning difficulties and a lack of concentration among pupils.

As far as the financial situation is concerned, although the majority of the population was able to manage its budget during this period, some people were affected by financial difficulties due to the loss of jobs.

The study was carried out over a short period of time, which means that other undesirable effects, which appear over the long term and may worsen with the age, history and risk factors of patients who have contracted Covid, should be anticipated.

Our work has given rise to the following perspectives

- Find the cause(s) of the prolonged symptoms: is viral persistence the rule or is it occasional? In which cells does the virus persist and what disturbances does it cause? What immunological, genetic, inflammatory or histological biomarkers characterise this prolonged infection?

- To evaluate interventions (pharmacological, psychological, rehabilitation) that have proved effective in other similar diseases, with a view to applying them in the case of Coronavirus.

- Identify new specific therapeutic and preventive interventions for these prolonged symptoms;

- Include Covid long patients and patient associations as partners in the research agenda and in the setting up of care structures, then ensure that these patients are properly monitored.

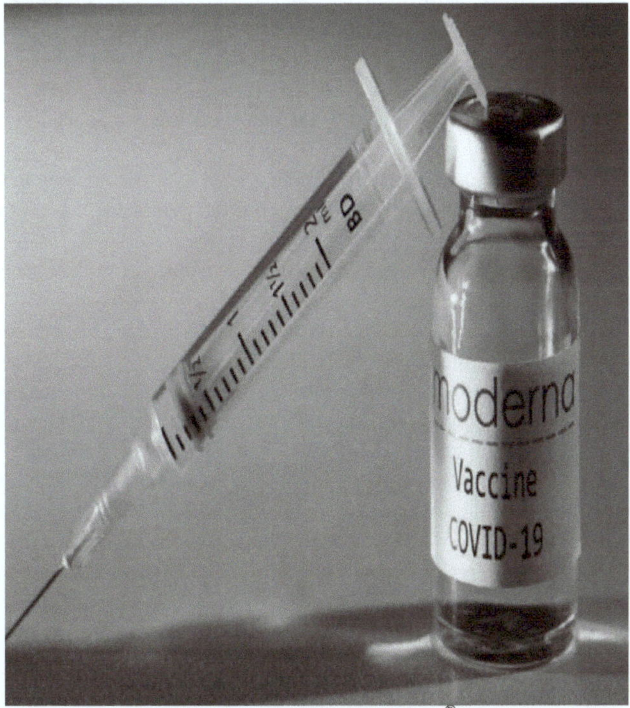

Figure 80. Example of Covid-19 vaccine, Moderna Spikevax[®].

References

1- Jie Cui, F. L.-L. (March 2019). Origin and evolution of pathogenic coronavirus. *Nature Review Microbiology.*

2- Ksiazek TG, E. D. (May 2003). A novel coronavirus associated with severe acute respiratory syndrome. *N Engl J Med.*

3- Zaki AM, v. B. (2012). Isolation of a novel coronavirus from a man with pneumonia in SaudiArabia.

4- Wong G, L. W. (2015). MERS, SARS, and Ebola: The role of super-spreaders in infection disease. *Cell Host Microbe.*

5- Guan Y, Z. B. (2003). Isolationd and characterizatioon of viruses related to the SARS corona-virus from animals in southern China. *Science.*

6- Azhar EI, E.-K. S.-S. (2014). Evidence for camel to human transmission of MERS coronavirus. *N Engl JMed.*

7- Zhu N, Z. D. (2020). A novel coronavirus from patients with pnneumonia in China 2019.

8- Wu Y, H. W. (2020). SARS-CoV-2 is an appropriate name for the new coronavirus. *Lancet.*

9- Li Q, G. X. (March 26, 2020). Early Transmission Dynamics in Wuhan, China, of Novel Coronavirus-Infected Pneumonia. *The new england joural of medicine.*

10- Okada P, B. R. (27 February 2020). Early transmission patterns of coronavirus disease 2019 (Covid-19) in travellers from Wuhan to Thailand.

11- *WHO.* (2020, January 12). who novel coronavirus (2019-nCov) situation report:https://www.who.int/emergencies/diseases/novel-coronavirus-2019/situation- reports.

12- China, Rëcupërë on WHO: https://covid19.who.int/region/wpro/country/cn

13- Li Yang Hsu, Po Ying Chia, Jeremy FY Lim (march 2020) Pandemic, T. N.- C.-2.

14- *WHO Director-General's opening remarks at the media briefing on COVID-19 - 11 March 2020.* (2020, march 11). WHO: https://www.who.int/director-general/speeches/detail/who-director-general-s-opening-remarks-at-the-media- briefing-on-covid-19 11-march-2020

15- *WHO Coronavirus (COVID-19) Dashboard* (2023).WHO: https://covid19.who.int/

16-(2023). Rëcupërë on our world in data: https://ourworldindata.org/explorers/coronavirus-data-explorer?zoomToSelection=true&time=2020-03-01.latest&facet=none&country=~DZA&pickerSort=desc&pickerMetric=location&Metric =Confirmed+cases&Interval=7 day+rolling+average&Relative+to+Population=true&Col 17- Gouilh, A. V. Coronavirus.

18- Caroline LEFEUVRE, E. P.-M. (October 2020). Virological aspects and diagnosis of Sars-CoV-2 coronavirus. *Actualites pharmaceutiques.*

19- Kannan S, S. S. (2020). COVID-19 (Novel Coronavirus 2019) - recent trends. *European Review for Medical and Pharmacological Sciences.*

20- Claude, J. *Covid-19.* Babelio: https://www.dev.scienceenlivre.org/covid-19/

21- Kiyotani, Y. T. (2020). SARS-CoV-2 genomic variations associated with mortality rate ofCOVID-19. *Journal of Human Genetics*, 1075-1082.

22- Alanagreh L, A. F. (2020). The Human Coronavirus Disease Covid- 19: Its Origin, Characteristics, and Insights into Potential Drugs and Its Mechanisms. *Pathogens.*

23- Jean-Daniel l.elievre, A. G.-D. (November 2020). Immunological and virological aspects of SARS-CoV-2 infection. *HAS.*

24- Muhammad Adnan Shereen, S. K. (2020). Covid-19 infection: Emergence, transmission, andcharacteristics of human coronaviruses. *Journal of Advanced Research*, 91-92.

25-Boni, M. L. (2020). Evolutionary origins of the SARS-CoV-2 sarbecovirus lineage responsible for the Covid-19 pandemic. *Nat Microbiol 5*, 1408-1417.

26-V. Bonny, A. M. (2020). Covid-19: pathophysiology of a multifaceted disease. *LaRevue deMedecine Interne,* 375-389.

27- Jianjian Wei PhD, Y. L. (2016). Airborne spread of infectious agents in the indoor environment. *American Journal of Infection Control.*

28- G. Birgand, S. K.-C. (2022). Modes of transmission of SARS-CoV-2: what is currently known? *Medecine et Maladies Infectieuses Formation*, 2-12.

29- Lingli Zhou, Z. X. (2020). ACE2 and TMPRSS2 are expressed on the human ocular surface,suggesting susceptibility to SARS-CoV-2 infection. *The Ocular Surface*, 537544.

30- Hasan K. Siddiqi, M. M. (2020). Covid-19 illness in native and immunosuppressed states: A clinical therapeutic staging proposal. *The journal of Heart and Lung Transplantation.*

31- Pericas JM, H.-M. M. (7 June 2020). Covid-19: from epidemiology to treatment. *European Heart Journal.*

32- Peiris S, M. H.-S. (April 2021). Pathological findings in organs and tissues of patients with Covid-19: A systematic review. *PLoS One.*

33- Polak SB, V. G. (November 2020). A systematic review of pathological findings in Covid-19: a pathophysiological timeline and possible mechanisms of disease progression. *Mod Pathol.*

34- Bach JF, B. P. (21 June 2021). Covid-19: individual and herd immunity. *C R Biol.*

35- Bakkouri, A. D. (2020). Current knowledge of 1 immunopathology of Covid-19. Revue marocaine de santë publique.

36- Blanco-Melo D, N.-P. B. (May 2021). mbalanced Host Response to SARS-CoV-2 Drives Development of Covid-19. *Cell.*

37- *Coronavirus and Covid-19 From the common cold to severe acute respiratory syndrome* (2022, May 12). INSERM: https://www.inserm.fr/dossier/coronavirus-sars-cov-et-mers-cov/

38- Abderrahmane, J. (2021). Enfants et Covid19: Expëгепсе de l'hopital тёге et enfant du CHU Mohammed VI de Marrakech. These pour l'obtention du Doctorat en Mëdecine. Faculte de Mëdecine et de Pharmacie Marrakech.

39- Sebastien Hantz, (November 2020). Biological diagnosis of Sars-CoV-2 infection: strategies and interpretation of results. *Rev Francoph Lab.*

40- N.Z.Lazli, L. F. (2020). Strategies therapeutiques dans la Covid-19 : revue de la litterature. *Revue Algerienne d'allergologie.*

41- Felsenstein S, H. J. (2020 June). Covid-19: Immunology and treatment options. *Clin Immunol.*

42- Hydroxychloroquine. Drug Bank: https://go.drugbank.com/drugs/DB01611

43- Hydroxychloroquine.   National Center for Biotechnology Information. PubChem:https://pubchem.ncbi.nlm.nih.gov/compound/hydroxychloroquine#section=   2D-Structure

44- Coronavirus 2019 (Covid-19): hydroxychloroquine (n.d.). World Health Organization: https://www.who.int/fr/news-room/questions-and-   answers/item/coronavirus-disease-(covid-

19)-hydroxychloroquine.

45- Satarker, S. A. (2020). Hydroxychloroquine in Covid-19: Potential Mechanism of Action Against SARS-CoV-2. *Curr Pharmacol Rep.*

46- *Chloroquine (1/2): The origin of quinine* (2020, May 02). Retrieved from Science trivia: https://www.citethisforme.com/cite/sources/websiteautociteeval

47- *Chloroquine.* Drug Bank: https://go.drugbank.com/drugs/DB00608

48- *Chloroquine.* PubChem: https://pubchem.ncbi.nlm.nih.gov/compound/2719

49- *The state of chloroquine consumption following its withdrawal.* Retrieved from Learn Online: https://www.clicours.com/etat-de-la-consommation-de-la-chloroquine-apres-son-withdrawal/ 50- Hawa, D. M. (n.d.). Les differentes strategies therapeutiques impliques dans le controle et le traitement de l'ëpidëmie Covie-19. Thëse pour l'obtention du diplôme de master.AbdelhafidBoussouf-Mila Departement des Sciences de la Nature et de la Vie.

51- HAS. (18 May 2020). Relatif a l'usage des anti-infectieux dans le Covid-19. 52- Durand, C. L. (2022). *DOROSZ Guide pratique des medicaments.* Maloine.53- Anthony C Moffat, M. D. (2011). *Clarke's Analysis of Drugs and Poisons.*

54- Damle B, V. M. (August 2020). Clinical Pharmacology Perspectives on the Antiviral Activity ofAzithromycin and Use in COVID-19. *Clin Pharmacol Ther.*

55-TRAORE Boubacar, T. B. (June 2020). COVID-19: Prise en charge therapeutique. Revue Marocaine de sante publique.

56- Bermejo-Martin JF, K. D. (April 2009). Macrolides for the treatment of severe respiratory illnesscaused by novel H1N1 swine influenza viral strains. *J Infect Dev Ctries.*

57- *Amoxicillin.* PubChem https://pubchem.ncbi.nlm.nih.gov/compound/amoxicil

58- *Beta-lactams | Structure | Mechanism of action | Spectrum of activity* (s.d.). Clinical microbiology: https://microbiologie-clinique.com/beta-lactamine.html

59- Comission de transparance, c. d. (16 february 2022). *tocilizumab,ROACTEMRA 20 mg/mL,* solution a diluer pour perfusion new indication.

60- Remdesivir. PubChem: https://pubchem.ncbi.nlm.nih.gov/compound/12130401661-Morse JS, L. T. (02 March 2020). Learning from the Past: Possible Urgent Prevention and Treatment Options for Severe Acute Respiratory Infections Caused by 2019-nCoV. *Chembiochem.*

62- National Center for Biotechnology Information. PubChem Compound Database: https://pubchem.ncbi.nlm.nih.gov/compound/Lopinavir- and- ritonavir

63- *KALETRA.* Vidal: https://www.vidal.fr/medicaments/gammes/kaletra-18372.html 64- HCSP. (23 July 2020). Rapport relatif a l'actualisation de la prise en charge des patients atteints de Covid-19.

65- Scientist, A. d. (2022, July 19). Covid-19, living with variants; the pandëmie is not over better anticipate.

66- *Nirmatrelvir.* PubChem: https://pubchem.ncbi.nlm.nih.gov/compound/Nirmatrelvir

67- Ferreira JC, R. W. (17 December 2020). Biochemical and biophysical characterization of the main protease, 3-chymotrypsin-like protease (3CLpro) from the novel coronavirus SARS-CoV-2. *Sci Rep.*

68- Rapid response in Covid-19, treatment with Paxlovid[®] for patients at risk of severe forms of Covid-19. (20 January 2020). *HAS.*

69-Yousra KHERABI, F.-X. L.-S. (2022). Covid-19: les therapeutiques. *Medecine et Maladies Infectieuses Formation*, 13-23.

70- WHO. (02 September 2020). Corticosteroids for the treatment of COVID-19.

71- *Cortisone and   corticoldes.* http://tice.ac-montpellier.fr/ABCDORGA/Family5/CORTICOIDS.htm

72- Covid-19 drug watch. (February 2021). *HAS.*

73- Dexamethasone KALCEKS 4mg/ 1 ml, injectable solution for infusion - Availability of a generic . (16 February 2022). *HAS.*

74- *Anakinra: Indication, Dosage, Side Effect, Precaution - MIMS Malaysia* (n.d.). rhttps://www.mims.com/malaysia/drug/info/anakinra

75- Covid-19: autorisation d'acces precoce accordee a un traitement prophylactique (s.d.). Haute Autorite De Sante.

76- ANSM, (2021, March). Therapeutic use and information collection protocol for Bamlanivimab and Etesevimab.

77- HAS. (August 2021). Ronapreve Solution to dilute for intravenous infusion or solution for subcutaneous injection.

78- Garrec, S. &. (1994). Paracetamol. Internat.

79- Mechanisms of action and toxicity of acetaminophen: clinical toxicology (s.d.). INSPQ: https://www.inspq.qc.ca/toxicologie-clinique/mecanismes-d-action-et-de-acetaminophen toxicity

80- Christophe Mallet, D. A. (2012). Paracëtamol: an ancestor with a future. *Therapies.*

81- Davenne E, G. J.-B. (2020). Coronavirus and Covid-19: an update on a rampant pandëmia. *RevMed Liege.*

82- Rothuizen, L. E. (2020). Treatments aggravating Covid-19 infection: really? *Rev Med Suisse.*

83- Pëters P, S. M. (2020). Coagulopathies, thrombotic risk and anticoagulation in Covid-19 . *Rev Med Liege.*

84- Couvreur, P., & Louvard, D. (2021). Covid-19 and drugs: pathophysiology and therapeuticapproaches. *Comptes Rendus. Biologies.*

85- *Vitamin D - Definition and Explanations.* (n.d.).Techno: https://www.techno-science.net/glossary-definition/Vitamin-D.html

86- Vitamin D and Covid-19. (2020). *Bulletin de l'Academie Nationale de Medecine.*

87- Naima Taqarort, S. C. (2020). Vitamin D and risk of acute respiratory infections: influenzaand Covid-19 . *Clinical Nutrition and Metabolism.*

88- *Molecular Structure Of Vitamin C by Greg Williams/science Photo Library.* (n.d.). Rëcupërë on Fine Art America: https://fineartamerica.com/featured/1-molecular- structure-of-vitamin-c-greg-williamsscience-photo-library.html

89- Komal, J. K. (2022). The role of vitamin C: From prevention of pneumonia to treatment of Covid-19. *Materials Today: Proceedings.*

90- Safieh Firouzi, N. P. (2022). The effect of Vitamin C and Zn supplementation on the immune system and clinical outcomes in COVID-19 patients. *Clinical Nutrition Open Science.*

91- Covid-19 vaccines: questions and answers. (29 dë December 2020). *SPILF.*

92- *List of   vaccines.* My vaccines.net: https://www.mesvaccins.net/web/vaccines?utf8=%E2%9C%93&name_or_disease=dis   eas e&searchby-name=&search-by-disease=57&commit=Chercher&search-by-age=&age_unit=years

93- Akrout, A. (2004). Etude des huiles essentielles de quelques plantes pastorales de la region de Matmata -Tunisie-.

94- Hasan A, B. P. (January 2020). Can Artemisia herba-alba Be Useful for Managing Covid-19 andComorbidities? *Molecules*.

95- *White wormwood* (2021, October 25). en.nina.az: https://www.wiki3.fr-en.nina.az/Armoise_herbe_blanche.html

96- *Thujone*. PubChem: https://pubchem.ncbi.nlm.nih.gov/compound/10931629

97-l.*8-Ciiieol-d3*. Rëcupërë on PubChem:

https://pubchem.ncbi.nlm.nih.gov/compound/4678102898- *Hispidulin*. PubChem: https://pubchem.ncbi.nlm.nih.gov/compound/5281628

99- MERRADI Massika, O. K. (2021). La guerissions a base de 1 Armoise blanche en medecine traditionnelle dans les Aures (Aigene) -Etude anthropologique-. *tributaries JOURNAL*.

100-OUIBRAHIM Amira (2015). Evaluation of the antimicrobial and antioxidant effect of three aromatic plants (Laurus nobilis L., Ocimumbasilicum L. and Rosmarinus officinalis L.) from EstAlgerien. Thëse pour l'obtention d'un diplôme de Doctoral (LMD). Faculte des sciences, Departement de Biologie.

101-Nabila Bourebaba, K. K.-G. (2021). Laurus nobilis ethanolic extract attenuates hyperglycemia and hyperinsulinemia-induced insulin resistance in HepG2 cell line through the reduction of oxidative stress and improvement of mitochondrial biogenesis - Possible implication inpharmacotherapy. *Mitochondrion*.

102-Ikram, B. F. (2021). Antimicrobial effects of the hydromdthanolic extract of Laurus nobilis L. on the growth of Staphylococus aureus. These pour l'obtention du diplôme de Masteren biologie. Laboratoire de microbiologie du département de biologie sise a la SNV-University of Mostaganem.

103-Siham Saleh Al-Abri, S. A.-S. (2022). Composition analysis and antimicrobial activity of essential oil from leaves of Laurus nobilis grown in Oman. *Journal of Bioresources and Bioproduct*.

104-Annelise Lobstein, F. C.-M. (2017). Laurel essential oil. *Actualites Pharmaceutiques*.

105-*Noble Laurel - Virtues, Benefits and Uses - Practical Guide* (2020, June 26). Doctonat: https://doctonat.com/laurier-noble/#usages-populaires

106-*Black Seed (Nigella sativa) seeds, organic* (s.d.). strictly medicinal seeds: https://strictlymedicinalseeds.com/product/black-seed-nigella-sativa-seeds-organic/

107-Tiwari, P. &. (2019). Nigella sativa: Phytochemistry, Pharmacology and its Therapeutic Potential. *Research Journal of Pharmacy and Technology*.

108-Eman R. Esharkawy, F. A. (2022). In vitro potential antiviral SARS-CoV-19- activity of natural product thymohydroquinone and dithymoquinone from Nigella sativa. *Bioorganic Chemistry*.

109-Khanna, T. F. (2017). CNS and analgesic studies on Nigella sativa. *Fitoterapia*.

110-Aljabre SHM, R. M. (2005). Antidermatophyte activity of ether extract of Nigella sativa and its active principle. *Journal of Ethnopharmacology*.

111-Anouar ABIDI, S. B. (2019). Pharmacological and physiological properties of Nigella Sativa L: Review of the literature. Revue FSB XVII 2019.

112-Ur Rehman, M. (2015). Nigella sativa: Monograph. *journal of pharmacognosy and phytochemistry*.

113-Shabir Ahmad Mir, A. F.-H. (2022). Identification of SARS-CoV-2 RNA-dependent RNA polymerase inhibitors from the major phytochemicals of Nigella sativa: An in silico approach. *Saudi Journal of Biological Sciences*.

114- What Is Nigella Sativa? Forms, Nutrients and Health Effects. Available at: https://www.healthline.com/nutrition/what-is-nigella-sativa

115- *What is eucalyptus globulus* (s.d.). Retrieved from Deiti Natura: https://www.dieti-natura.com/active-plants/eucalyptus-globulus.html/

116- *alpha-PINENE*. PubChem: https://pubchem.ncbi.nlm.nih.gov/compound/alpha- pinene

117- Hayat, U. &. (2015). A Review on Eucalyptus globulus: A New Perspective in Therapeutics. 118- Eucalyptus : ou le planter, entretien, multiplier (04/05/2022) Recupere sur le journal desfemmes : https://www.j ournaldesfemmes.fr/jardin/encyclopedie-des-plantes/2404698-eucalyptus/#:~:text=Ses%20fleurs%2C%20qui%20apparaissent%20au%20printemps%20ou%20e n,g%C3%A9n%C3%A9ralement%20comme%20huile%20essentielle%20pour%20d%C3%A9ga ger%20les%20bronches.

119- *Clove: 208,591 images, photos and stock vector images*. (n.d.). Shutter Stock: https://www.shutterstock.com/fr/search/clou-de-girofle

120- *Clove*. (2017, January 27). Doctissimo: https://www.doctissimo.fr/html/sante/phytotherapie/plante-medicinal/girofle.htm#composition-du-girofle

121- Iserin, P. (s.d.). *Encyclopaedia of medicinal plants*. La Rousse.

122- *Eugenol*. PubChem: https://pubchem.ncbi.nlm.nih.gov/compound/eugenol

123- *Cloves: properties, benefits and contraindications*. (2022, January 21). Hospital information: Medical lexicon and news: https://www.informationhospitaliere.com/clou-de-girofle-proprietes-bienfaits-et-contraindications

124- National Institute for Health and Care Excellence (NICE), R. C. (2020). *COVID-19 Rapid Guideline: Managing the Long-Term Effects of Covid-19*. National Institutefor Health and Care Excellence: https://www.nice.org.uk/guidance/ng188

125- HAS. (2021). Symptoms prolongës suite a Covid-19 de l'adulte - Diagnostic et prise encharge.

126- Activated charcoal, a lead against long forms of Covid (13 June 2021). Rëponses Bio: https://www.reponsesbio.com/le-charbon-active-une-piste-contre-les- long-form-covid/

127- L Carl Brown, A. E. (2023). *Algerie. Britannica* https://www.britannica.com/place/Algeria

128- William G. Smith, P. (2008). Does Gender Influence Online Survey Participation? ARecord-linkage Analysis of University Faculty.

129- Underwood, D., Kim, H., & Matier, M. (2000). To Mail or To Web: Comparisons of SurveyResponse Rates and Respondent Characteristics. AIR 2000 Annual Forum Paper.

130- WHO reveals the main causes of death and disability in the world: 2000-2019. (2020). WHO.

131- *Statistics on the spread of the Corona virus in Algeria*. elaph: https://elaph.com/coronavirus-statistics-in-algeria.html

132- *WHO. Monitoring of SARS-CoV-2 variants* (2023, 3 30). WHO: https://www.who.int/fr/activities/tracking-SARS-CoV-2-variants

133- Xiangying Ren, J. Z. (2022, April 22). *Reinfection in patients with CO VID-19: a systematic review*. Springer link: https://link.springer.com/article/10.1186/s41256- 022-

00245-3

134- Faucherb, E. D.-F. (2020). Covid-19: clinical aspects and main elements of management. *Revue francophone des laboratoires*.

135- Ali Nadi, A. A. (2023). Thymus vulgaris, a natural pharmacy against Covid-19: Amolecular review. *Journal of Herbal Medicine*.

136- Ammar, A. (08/2022). Acceptability of the Covid-19 vaccine in the Tunisian population. *Revue d'Epidemiologie et de Sante Publique*.

137- Alsahali, A. (2021, 9 29). *Algerie demarre sa production de vaccins contre le Covid-19.*

RFI: https://www.rfi.fr/fr/afrique/20210929-l-alg%C3%A9rie-d%C3%A9marre-sits-production-of-vaccines-against-covid-19

138- *Coronavirus vaccines: more than a billion doses injected worldwide.* (n.d.). on HuffPost: https://www.huffingtonpost.fr/actualites/article/vaccins-contre-le-coronavirus-more-than-a-billion-doses-injected-around-the-world_180375.html

139-Pfizer; Sinopharm, Sputnik V... Which vaccines are used worldwide!

cnews: https://www.cnews.fr/monde/2021-02-01/pfizer-sinopharm-sputnik-v-what-vaccines-are-used-around-the-world-1041720

140- Adverse reactions to vaxzevria vaccine (ASTRAZENECA). (January 2023). *ANSM*

141- *The* World Health Organisation publishes a definition of post-Covid-19 disease to aid treatment. Retrieved from United Nations: https://news.un.org/fr/story/2021/10/1105862

142- Dominique SALMON CERON, B. D. (2022). Prolonged forms of COVID-.

19 orCOVID long: clinical forms and management. *Medecine et Maladies Infectieuses Formation*.

143- SeeBle Jessica, W. T. (1 April 2022). Persistent Symptoms in Adult Patients 1 Year After Coronavirus Disease 2019 (COVID-19): A Prospective Cohort Study. *Clinical InfectiousDiseases*.

144- *Prolonged symptoms following adult Covid-19 - Diagnosis and management* .(2021, february 12). Haute autorite de sante: https://www.has-sante.fr/icms/p 3237041/en/symptomes-prolonges-suite-a-a-covid-19-de-l-adulte-diagnostic-et-prise-en-charge

145- WHO. (2021, March 26). *Latest information on the long-term clinical effects of Covid-19.*

146- Ceron, D. S. (2021, November 19). Actualites sur les aspects cliniques du Covid long *Colloque Spilf sur le Covid long*.

147- HAS. (2021). Neurological manifestations among the prolonged symptoms of Covid-19.

148- Arnold D.T., H. F. (2021). The Writing Committee for the COMEBAC Study Group Four- Month Clinical Status of a cohort of patients after hospitalization for COVID- 19. JAMA.

149- Huang C., H. L. 6-month consequences of COVID-19 in patients dischargedfrom hospital: a cohort study. Lancet. 2021 . 220-232.

150- Groff D., S. A. (2021). *PubMed Central (PMC)*. Recupere on Short-term and Longterm rates of postacute sequelae of SARS-CoV-2 infection. A systematic review. JAMA NetwOpen.2021; available at: https://www.ncbi.nlm.nih.gov/pmc/articles/PMC9122778/

151- CHERET, D. S. (2021). *Societe depathologie infectieuse de langue franqaise (SPILF).*

https://doi.org/10.1016Zj.mmifmc.2021.12.001

152-   Stahlberg M, R. U. (2021). *Post-Covid-19 tachycardia syndrome: distinct phenotype from post-acute Covid-19 syndrome. Am J Med.*

153-   Yan Xie, Evan Xu, Benjamin Bowe & Ziyad Al-Aly 07 February 2022 Nature Medicinevolume available at: https://www.nature.com/articles/s41591-022- 01689-3

154-   *Digestive symptoms among the symptoms of Covid-19.* (2023, January 19). www.has-sante.fr

155-   Joint pain: symptoms after Covid available on: rafael postcovid.ch

156-   *Report-on-Long-Covid-Impact-Survey* (2021, June 08).
https://imgix.cosmicjs.com/d8d3d3b0-c936-11eb-ba89-e7f98c8c358b-FINAL—   Report-on-T.ong-Covid-Impact-Survey—June-8-2021 pdf

157-   Meloche-Holubowski, M. (n.d.). *What do we know about post-Covid-19 syndrome? Coronavirus* Radio-Canada.ca

158- *covid   long   a   sometimes   disabling   disease.* (2022).   valwin.fr:
https://valwin.fr/blog/20220216-le-covid-long-une-maladie-parfois disabling/?pharmacyId=undefined)

159-   Li X., X. S. (2020). *Risk factors for severity and mortality in adult* Covid-19 *inpatients in Wuhan. Allergy Clin Immunol.*

160-   SULLIVAN, B. (2021, June 14). Can Covid-19 cause diabetes?
? National Geographic

161-Nanki Hura BS, D. X. (2020, June 22). https://doi.org/10.1002/alr.22624 162- al., D. S. (2021, novombre). *Actualites sur les aspects cliniques du COVID long -Clinical, virological and imaging profile in patients with Persistent or resurgent forms of COVID- 19: a cross-sectional study. J Infection-universite de paris.*

163-Cristina   Menni,   P.   *.   (2022,   April   07).   DOI:https: //doi.org/10.1016/S0140-6736(22)00327-0.

164-Philippe Ornell, S. C. (2020). scielo - the impact of the Covid-19 pandemicon the mental health of healthcare professionals 2020: https://doi.org/10.1590/0102- 311X00063520

165-David Montani, a. L.-M.-L.-F. (2023, April 25). *post covid syndrome.* Retrieved from PubMedCentral: https://www.nvbi.nlm.nih.gov/pmc/articles/PMC10126882/

166-Maude Dionne, E. D. (2021, July 23). *institut national de sante publique du quebec* . inspq.qc.ca:
https://www.google.com/url?sa=t&source=web&rct=j&url=https://www.inspq.qc.ca/si   tes/ default/files/publications/3149-pandemie-impact-life-
personal.pdf&ved=2ahUKEwihmrrnkoz AhXsy7sIHW78BO8QFnoECAgQAQ&u sg= AOvVaw0dAkd4OgmfY8ImQr9tWroL

167-Salmon-Ceron, D. e. (2021). *Clinical, virological and imaging profile in patients with prolonged forms of Covid-19: A cross-sectional study. J Infect, 2021.*

168-Tremblay, D.-G. e. (2020). *Prospects for the future of work: Telework, coworking and other third places. In A. Gillet, ed.* Travailler dans les services publics : la nouvelle donne. Paris: Presses de l'EHESP. p. 139-146.

169-alberio, M. *Covid-19, the effects on work and employment.*
https://joumals.openedition.org/interventionseconomiques/14725)

Appendices

Survey form

Survey on the impact of 1 Coronavirus infection on the Algerian population Sequelles organiques et psycho-sociales.

Part I: Data relating to the subjects.

Partie I : Données relatives aux sujets.

-Sexe : ☐ Masculin ☐ Féminin

-Age : ☐ < 18 ☐ [18-30[☐ [30-50[☐ Plus de 50 ans

-Wilaya :..............

-Niveau d'étude : ☐ Non scolarisé(e) ☐ Primaire ☐ Moyen ☐ Secondaire ☐ Universitaire

-Situation sociale : ☐ Marié ☐ Célibataire

-Quelle est votre catégorie socioprofessionnelle ?

☐ Étudiant(e) ☐ Fonctionnaire ☐ Sans emploi ☐ Commerçant(e) ☐ Retraité

-Souffrez-vous d'une maladie chronique ? ☐ Oui ☐ Non

Si oui ; la(les)quelle(s) ?

☐ Diabète ☐

☐ Maladie cardiovasculaire (insuffisance ☐

cardiaque, HTA....) ☐

☐ Insuffisance rénale ☐

☐ Insuffisance hépatique

☐ Maladie respiratoire (asthme...)

Partie II : Infection au Sars-CoV-2.

-Avez-vous déjà attrapé la Covid ? ☐ Oui   ☐ Non   Thyroïdites
                         ☐   ☐   Polyarthrite rhumatoïde
                                                          Maladie cœliaque
                                                          Cancer
                                                          Autre :……

Si oui, combien de fois ?   Une seule fois   Deux fois   Plus de deux fois
                                                        ☐

-Quel(s) symptôme(s) ou signe(s) de la maladie avez-vous eu ?
   ☐ De la fièvre.   ☐ Le nez qui coule.
   ☐ Des maux de tête.   ☐ Des difficultés respiratoires (difficultés
   ☐ Des courbatures.   importantes à respirer, essoufflements…)
   ☐ De la toux.   ☐ Une perte de l'odorat ou du goût.
   ☐ Des diarrhées.   ☐ De la fatigue.
   ☐ Des douleurs au ventre.   ☐ Asphyxie
   ☐ Des maux de gorge.   -Autre :……

-Combien de temps ont duré vos symptômes ?
        ☐   ☐   ☐   ☐
☐1-5jrs   6-10jrs   11-15 jrs   16-20 jrs   Plus que 20jrs   Je ne sais pas
                                                                     ☐

-Y a-t-il, dans votre entourage ou votre famille, des personnes qui ont eu le Coronavirus ou des signes de
maladie laissant à penser que c'était le Coronavirus (Covid-19) ?   ☐ Oui   ☐Non
-Vous a-t-on fait un test pour savoir si c'était le Coronavirus (Covid-19) ?   ☐ Oui   ☐Non
Si oui ; lequel ?   ☐Test PCR   ☐Test sérologique   ☐Test antigénique
-Avez-vous consulté un médecin ou été hospitalisé suite à ces symptômes de la maladie ?
   ☐Oui, j'ai consulté un médecin   ☐Oui, j'ai été hospitalisé(e)   ☐ Non

-veuillez sélectionner le type de traitement médicamenteux que vous avez pris ?
   ☐Aucun
   ☐Hydroxychloroquine, Chloroquine   lopinavir+nirmatrelvir) Corticoïdes
   ☐ Antibiotiques (azithromycine,   (hydrocortisone, dexaméthasone, prednisone..)
      amoxicilline…)
   ☐ Antiviraux (remdesivir,   Autre: ………

-Avez-vous utilisé des plantes médicinales lors du traitement ?   ☐ Oui   Non
Si oui la (les) quelle (s) ?

   ☐ L'armoise blanche   ☐ L'eucalyptus   ☐ Le gingembre
   ☐ Le thym   ☐ Le laurier noble   ☐ Le clou de girofleالقرنفل
   ☐ La menthe   ☐ La Nigelle cultivée   Autre : ………
   ☐ La verveine   ☐ Le Romarin
                                    ☐
-Avez-vous reçu le vaccin contre la Covid-19 ?   Oui   ☐Non
Si oui, quel type de vaccin avez-vous reçu ?
   ☐Vaxzevria (Astrazeneca)   ☐Spikevax (Moderna)
   ☐Sputnik V (Gamelya)   ☐Comernaty (Pfizer-bioNtech)
   ☐Coronavac (Sinovac)   ☐Je ne sais pas

Vitamine et suppléments minéraux(vitamine C, D, zinc…) ☐

Part III : les séquelles organiques et psycho-sociales de Sars-CoV-2

1. Séquelles organiques :

-Après la première semaine vos symptômes ont-ils ? ☐ Régressés ☐ Aggravés

-Après combien de jours avez-vous été guéri complètement ?

☐1-5jrs ☐6-10jrs ☐11-15jrs ☐16-20jrs ☐21-25jrs ☐26-30jrs ☐Plus que 30jrs

-Avez-vous encore aujourd'hui ces symptômes ou signes de la maladie ? ☐Oui ☐Non

-si oui le(s)quel(s) :

Type de symptômes :		Oui	Non
Symptômes généraux	Fatigue		
	Obésité		
	Perte de poids		
Symptômes neurologiques	Epilepsie		
	Troubles de sommeil		
	Céphalées		
	Vertiges		
	Troubles de mémoire		
Symptômes respiratoires	Dyspnée		
	BPCO		
	Asthme		
	Hyperactivité bronchique		
Symptômes cardiovasculaires	HTA		
	Insuffisance cardiaque		
	Arythmie		
Symptômes digestifs	Gastrite ou œsophagite		
	Diarrhée		
	Constipation		
	Douleurs abdominales		
Symptômes musculo-tendineux et articulaires	Myalgie		
	Douleurs articulaires		
Symptômes oculaires	Diminution de l'acuité visuelle		
	Douleur oculaire		
	Fatigue visuelle		
Symptômes endocriniens	Diabète		
	Thyroïdite		
Autre :	Coagulopathie		
	Insuffisance rénale		

1. Séquelles psychiques

-Avant la Covid, avez-vous souffert d'un (des) trouble (s) psychique (s) ? ☐ Oui ☐ Non
-Pendant la Covid, avez-vous souffert d'un (des) trouble (s) psychiatrique (s) ? ☐ Oui ☐ Non
Si oui, le(s)quel(s) :

☐ Anxiété	☐ Dépression
☐ Irritabilité	☐ Phobie
☐ Manque de concentration	☐ Trouble obsessionnelle compulsif
☐ Nervosité	☐ Schizophrénie
☐ Trouble de panique	Autre :…………

-Pendant la Covid, avez-vous pris des médicaments pour traiter des problèmes neurologiques (hypnotiques, tranquillisants, ou des antidépresseurs) ? ☐ Oui ☐ Non
-Avez-vous aujourd'hui des symptômes psychiques suite au période d'épidémie Covid19 ?
☐ Oui ☐ Non
Si oui le(s)quel(s) :

☐ Anxiété	☐ Trouble de panique
☐ Irritabilité	☐ Phobie
☐ Manque de concentration	☐ Trouble obsessionnelle compulsif
☐ Nervosité	Autre :…………
☐ Dépression	

2. Séquelles sociales

-Avez-vous arrêté vos activités quotidiennes à cause de Covid ? ☐ Oui ☐ Non
-Avez-vous arrêté le travail à cause de Covid 19 ? ☐ Temporairement ☐ Définitivement ☐ Non
Si définitivement, avez-vous trouvé un autre travail ? ☐ Oui ☐ Non
Si oui, dans quel domaine : ☐ Télétravail (freelance) ☐ Étatique ☐ Privé
-Avez-vous arrêté votre éducation à cause de Covid 19 ? ☐ Oui ☐ Non
-

☐ Ça va
☐ Vous y arrivez difficilement
☐ Vous ne pouvez pas y arriver sans faire de dettes.

-Quel est l'impact de Covid sur votre situation familiale : ☐ Sans impact ☐ Mariage ☐ Divorce
-Si vous étiez mariés avant la Covid, avez-vous eu des enfants ? ☐ ☐

**Investigation on the impact of the Coronavirus infection on the
Algerian population : organic and psychosocial sequalae.**

Fiche d'enquete (version anglaise)

Part I: Subject data

-Sex: ☐Male ☐Female

-Age: ☐<18 ☐[18-30[☐[30-50] ☐>50

-The state: ....

-Level of study:

☐out of school ☐primary school ☐middle school ☐secondary school ☐university

-Social status: ☐married ☐single

-What is your socio-professional category: ☐student ☐employed ☐jobless ☐retired

-Do you suffer from a chronic disease? ☐Yes ☐No

-if yes, which one(s)?

☐Diabetes ☐Thyroiditis

☐Cardiovascular disease (heart failure, hypertension…) ☐Rheumatoid arthritis

☐Renal insufficiency ☐Celiac disease ☐Cancer

☐Hepatic insufficiency Other: …

☐Respiratory disease (asthma…)

Part II: Sras-CoV-2 infection

-Have you ever infected with Covid? ☐Yes ☐no

If yes, how many times? ☐Once ☐twice ☐more than twice

-What symptom(s) or sign(s) of the disease did you have?

☐Fever ☐Runny nose

☐Headaches ☐Breathing difficulties (shortness of breath…..)

☐Aches and pain

☐Coughing ☐Loss of smell or taste

☐Diarrhoea ☐Fatigue

☐Belly pain ☐Asphyxia

☐Sore throat Other: ….

-How long did your symptoms last? …….. days ☐I don't know

-Has any of your family felt symptoms of corona or did he get sick of it? ☐Yes ☐No

-Have you taken a corona test to make sure you are sick? ☐Yes ☐No

If yes, which one? ☐ PCR test ☐Serological test ☐Antigenic test

-Have you consulted a doctor or been hospitalized because of symptoms of coronavirus?

☐Yes, I saw a doctor ☐Yes, I was hospitalized ☐No

-Please select the type of medication you have been taken?

☐None

☐Hydroxychloroquine, chloroquine

☐Antibiotics (azithromycin, amoxicillin…)

☐Antiviral (remdesivir, lopinavir+nirmatrelvir…)

☐Corticosteroids (prednisone, hydrocortisone, dexamethasone…)

☐Analgesics (paracetamol…)

-Did you use medicinal herbs during the treatment?

If so, which one(s)?

Antihistamines (loratadine, dexchloropheniramine…) ☐Vitamin and mineral supplements (vitamin C, vitamin D, Zinc…)

Anticoagulants (enoxaparin…) ☐Other: ….

Antitussives (pholcodine, dextromethorphan…) ☐Yes ☐ No

Throat spray (Hexaspray®, Humex®…) ☐

☐White wormwood Eucalyptus ☐ Ginger

☐Thyme Laurus nobilis Clove

☐Mentha Nigella sativa Other: …

☐Vervain Rosemary

-Have you received the Covid vaccine?　　☐Yes　　　☐No
-if yes, which one?
　　☐Vaxzevria (Astrazeneca)　　　　　　☐Spikevax (Moderna)
　　☐Sputnik V (Gamelya)　　　　　　　　☐Comernaty (Pfizer-bioNtech)
　　☐Coronavac (Sinovac)　　　　　　　　☐I don't know

Part III: the organic and psychosocial sequalae of Sras-CoV-2

1. Organic sequalae:

-After the first week, did your symptoms?　　☐ Regressed　☐ Aggravated
-After how many days did you recover?
☐1-5　　☐6-10　　☐11-15　　☐16-20　☐21-25　　☐26-30　☐More than 30days
-Do you still feel these symptoms?　　☐Yes　☐No
If yes, which one(s)?

Type of symptoms:		Yes	No
General symptoms	Tiredness		
	Obesity		
	Weight loss		
Neurological symptoms	Epilepsy		
	Sleep disorder		
	Headaches		
	Dizziness		
	Memory disorder		
Pulmonary symptoms	Dyspnoea		
	CPOD		
	Asthma		
	Bronchial hyperactivity		
Cardiovascular symptoms	Hypertension (HBP)		
	Heart failure		
	Arrythmia		
Digestive symptoms	Gastritis or oesophagitis		
	Diarrhoea		
	Constipation		
	Abdominal pain		
Musculo-tendinous and articular Symptoms	Myalgia		
	Joint pain		
Ocular symptoms	Decreased visual acuity		
	Eye pain		
	Visual fatigue		
Endocrine symptoms	Diabetes		
	Thyroiditis		
Other	Coagulopathy		
	Renal insufficiency		

2. Psychic sequelae:

-Before Covid, have you suffered from any psychiatric disorder?   ☐ Yes   ☐ No
-During Covid, have you suffered from any psychiatric disorder?   ☐ Yes   ☐ No
If yes, which one(s)?

☐ Anxiety   ☐ Panic disorder
☐ Phobia   ☐ Depression
☐ Irritability   ☐ Obsessive-compulsive disorder
☐ Lack of concentration   ☐ Schizophrenia
☐ Nervousness   Other: …

-During Covid, have you taken any medications to treat neurological problems (hypnotics, tranquilizers or antidepressants)?   ☐ Yes   ☐ No
-Do you have today any psychological symptoms as a result of Covid-19 epidemic?   ☐ Yes ☐ No
If yes, which one(s)?

☐ Anxiety   ☐ Depression
☐ Phobia   ☐ Obsessive-compulsive disorder
☐ Irritability   ☐ Schizophrenia
☐ Lack of concentration   Other: …
☐ Nervousness
☐ Panic disorder

3. Social sequalae:

-Have you stopped your daily activities because of Covid-19? ☐ Yes   ☐ No
-Have you stopped working because of Covid-19? ☐ No   Temporarily ☐ Definitely
If definitely, have you found another job?   ☐ Yes   ☐ No

If yes, in which field?   Teleworking (freelance) ☐ Yes ☐ Public   ☐ Private

-Did you stop your education because of Covid-19?   ☐ No
-During Covid-19, financially:
☐ You were comfortable   ☐   you could hard do it
☐ ☐ ☐ ☐

What is the impact of Covid-19 on your familial status?
If you get married before Covid, did you have children

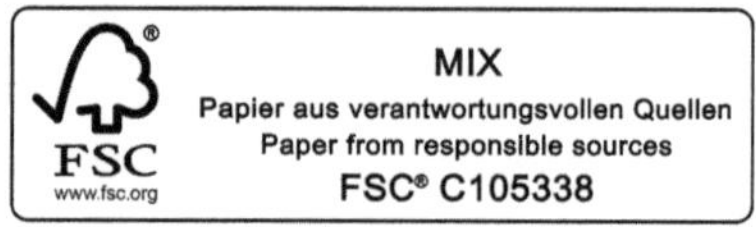

Printed by Books on Demand GmbH, Norderstedt / Germany